essential tremor

the facts

also available in the series

essential tremor

the facts

DR MARK PLUMB
Senior Lecturer, Department of Genetics,
University of Leicester, UK

DR PETER BAIN
Reader and Honorary Consultant in Clinical Neurology,
University Department of Clinical Neurosciences,
Imperial College London, UK

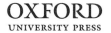
OXFORD
UNIVERSITY PRESS

OXFORD
UNIVERSITY PRESS

Great Clarendon Street, Oxford OX2 6DP

Oxford University Press is a department of the University of Oxford.
It furthers the University's objective of excellence in research, scholarship,
and education by publishing worldwide in

Oxford New York

Auckland Cape Town Dar es Salaam Hong Kong Karachi
Kuala Lumpur Madrid Melbourne Mexico City Nairobi
New Delhi Shanghai Taipei Toronto

With offices in

Argentina Austria Brazil Chile Czech Republic France Greece
Guatemala Hungary Italy Japan Poland Portugal Singapore
South Korea Switzerland Thailand Turkey Ukraine Vietnam

Oxford is a registered trade mark of Oxford University Press
in the UK and in certain other countries

Published in the United States
by Oxford University Press Inc., New York

British Library Cataloguing in Publication Data
Data available

Library of Congress Cataloging in Publication Data
Data available

Typeset by Newgen Imaging Systems (P) Ltd., Chennai, India
Printed in Great Britain
on acid-free paper by
Clays Ltd., Bungay, Suffolk

ISBN 978–0–19–921127–2 (Pbk: alk paper)

1

contents

preface

Essential tremor (ET) affects a very large number of people worldwide, all of whom have a right to up-to-date information on this disorder which affects their lives and those of their partners and families. We feel that this access to information about ET is a basic human right. Whilst many may not be particularly interested, affected and unaffected individuals (and their families) should at least have the facility to access current information about essential tremor in a comprehensible form, if they so wish.

The biology underlying ET is not fully understood, although significant progress is being made. In fact, a large amount of very exciting scientific and clinical information is now available. The ability of science to describe in some detail how an electrical signal is generated inside a single nerve cell and is then transmitted to another is a spectacular achievement, and also provides an intriguing glimpse at the machinery that makes a human mind. Similarly, the scientific journey which starts with a few ET families and will one day soon result in the identification of the gene(s) that causes ET is equally interesting and is a good illustration of the logical and technical processes researchers employ to understand inherited diseases.

The main aim of this book is to bring together all that information in one place, in a readable form. Some interesting ideas have emerged consequent to the book's development. The authors hope that this information will significantly help people to understand, live and cope with ET, and also help raise awareness of ET across society.

The study of ET is a complex multidisciplinary subject about a condition that affects many aspects of people and society. It is a disorder of the central nervous system's regulatory circuits which control voluntary movement. The basic principles underlying ET are gradually becoming understood and it is already possible to predict to some degree both the likely causes of the disorder and the key future research avenues. Other neurological problems relate in complex ways to this disorder, and the relationship of anxiety to ET is a central theme of this book. There is at present no cure for ET, but medication is available to suppress symptoms. How that medication works and the potential side effects are important both for the patient who is being treated and also for our understanding of the causes of ET. Currently, very promising strategies are being explored in Parkinson's disease and other movement disorders which may eventually prove applicable to ET. With luck, key breakthroughs in the understanding of ET and its treatment are not too far away.

Dr Mark Plumb is a qualified Biochemist (BSc, PhD) specializing in cancer genetics. His professional scientific research career has focused on the causes of leukaemia. However, he has been affected by ET since he was an infant, has a large family that is affected by ET, and has spent the last 5 years researching the available peer-reviewed literature on ET. It is the fruits of this research, and his personal experiences, that form the backdrop to this book.

Dr Peter Bain is a Reader in Clinical Neurology at Imperial College London, and practises as a consultant neurologist. He runs specialized movement disorder and tremor clinics at Charing Cross Hospital, London. He has been actively involved in tremor research for more than 10 years, and has written over 150 articles on essential and various other types of tremor and movement disorders. He has a particular interest in the classification, diagnosis, measurement methodology, and medical and surgical treatment of tremor, including deep brain stimulation, and hopes that this knowledge will benefit those who suffer from ET.

MP & PB

foreword by Professor Leslie J Findley

Essential tremors (ET) represent the commonest disorders of movement seen in man. A conservative estimate would state that at least 600,000 people in the UK are affected with ET. These disorders represent a largely unappreciated and sizeable source of national morbidity, being many times more common than some of the better known movement disorders, such as Parkinson's disease and dystonia.

On the basis of the aphorism "knowledge dispels fear" it is appropriate that this volume in "The Facts" series is dedicated to this group of disorders.

The authors are each singularly qualified in their own way to offer this volume to us. Dr Peter Bain is a world leader in the scientific and clinical investigations of ET, whereas Dr Mark Plumb is not only a world renowned scientist, but has the distinction of being one of the few authors in this series to have personal experience of the condition he is describing.

This concise monograph presents, with clarity, the current understanding and limits of knowledge of ET, in a format which will be readily appreciated by those with tremors. The authors describe and emphasize areas of concern, which have often been avoided in standard clinical texts, eg areas of lack of basic knowledge, social and emotional effects of ET, low awareness in the population, paucitiy and limitation of treatments available etc.

The background physiology, genetics and epidemiology are presented in a way in which the lay person will appreciate and understand. However, I think the non specialist clinicians and other health professionals will find this volume a source of readily available facts in a digestible form. The authors probe state of the art current treatments, as well as discuss the place of, or otherwise, the modern technology such as gene therapies and stem cells.

This volume was a pleasure to read. I am sure it is going to be welcomed enthusiastically by members of the tremor support charities, as a valuable source of intelligible information

Professor Leslie J Findley
Consultant Neurologist, Essex Neurosciences Unit
Chairman, Board of Trustees, National Tremor Foundation (UK)

foreword by Mark Hallett, M.D.

Essential tremor is one of the most common afflictions of humans, affecting about 1 out of every 100 persons. Yet it is often not recognized, often misdiagnosed, not well treated, and not fully understood. Thus, it is important to get the Facts out to the public to increase awareness and understanding of the situation. Doctors can help, but patients do need to take some control of their health. In relation to recognition and diagnosis, there are many different types of tremor, so it does take some expertise to make the correct identification of essential tremor. When mild, sometimes even the experts have trouble being sure. When very mild, some patients don't even recognize that they have a problem; they might consider a slight tremor just "normal" or perhaps just something that many other persons in the family have. In regard to treatment, there are some medications that can provide benefit, and some patients have not had the opportunity to try them. For severe cases, brain surgery can provide excellent benefit and this is likely not as widely used as it might be. But, in general, we need more work in developing better therapies. In relation to further research needed, we still need to understand exactly how the brain generates the tremor. Since essential tremor is often genetic, progress in genetics, a hot area, may well help. Better understanding should lead to new approaches to therapy. This book, written by experts, presents current knowledge in all these areas in a very readable form. It should be helpful to anyone seeking information about essential tremor.

Mark Hallett, M.D.

acknowledgements

The authors would particularly like to express their gratitude and admiration to all the affected and unaffected individuals who volunteered for the clinical and scientific studies of ET. They have, and continue to make, an invaluable contribution to the progress being made in understanding the causes and treatments of this movement disorder.

The authors would also like to thank everyone that helped during the preparation of this manuscript and contributed their personal perspectives. In particular David Tomley, Gill Thomas, Anita Harmer, and Claire and Katie Plumb.

Whilst every effort has been made to ensure that the contents of this book are as complete, accurate, and up to date as possible at the date of writing, Oxford University Press is not able to give any guarantee or assurance that such is the case. Readers are urged to take appropriately qualified medical advice in all cases. The information in this book is intended to be useful to the general reader, but should not be used as a means of self-diagnosis or for the prescription of medication.

1 What is essential tremor?

The main characteristic of essential tremor (ET) is shaking of the hands, although shaking can also affect the head, voice, face and legs. This is most easily illustrated by the difficulty affected individuals have in writing or drawing a spiral, as illustrated in Fig. 1.1.

ET is one of many different causes of tremor and is not a simple disorder. In this chapter, we will review the particular characteristics of the ET tremor, namely *postural* and *kinetic* tremor, and consider some of the other criteria used to define ET.

There is also increasing evidence that psychological stress makes ET much worse. The technical words to describe this include *sociophobia*, *harm avoidance*, and *psychosocial dysfunction*. However, these terms describe a person who avoids interacting with society, and in ET this can be reduced to self-conscious embarrassment. Throughout this book, we will argue that this anxious personality trait is part and parcel of ET, and in many cases has a much greater effect on living than the tremor itself.

The first step is to understand the terms 'postural' and 'kinetic' tremor.

- Postural tremor occurs when part of the body is held against gravity such as holding the arms in front of the body (both arms usually shake, bilateral tremor) or holding the head still.

- Kinetic tremor is also called action tremor and is observed during voluntary movement such as writing, drawing, pouring, etc.

Most importantly, ET does not occur at rest. Even in severely affected people, if the muscles are completely relaxed, no tremor will be detected, and people with ET do not shake when they are fast asleep.

Other key characteristics of ET which have been well documented include the following

- Variable tremor severity.

- A tendency for the symptoms to worsen during emotional and physical stress.

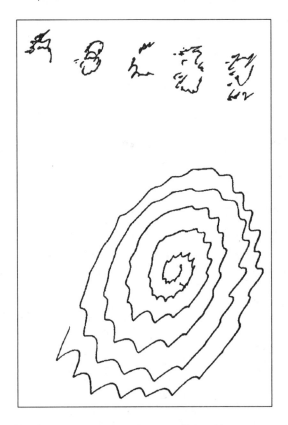

Figure 1.1 Spirograph/writing in ET. The postural and kinetic tremor in ET during voluntary movement in the arms, wrists and fingers is well illustrated in the difficulties with writing and drawing a spiral (spirography).

- A tendency for the symptoms to worsen with age.
- A variable age of onset, including childhood.
- ET often runs in families.
- ET can be *sporadic—there* are some cases of ET with no obvious family history. This suggests that environmental factors may play a causal role, although precisely which environmental factor(s) are involved is unknown.

ET is thus a very complex and *heterogenous* disorder. So that, except for the presence of the characteristic postural and kinetic tremor, everything else in ET is highly variable: severity; age of onset; family history (*genetics*); and other 'symptoms', all exhibit tremendous interindividual variation, both in ET populations as a whole and also within individual families. The use of the word 'complex' in this context simply means that the disorder is not fully understood.

In this and subsequent chapters, we will build up a picture of ET, and although the precise neurological defect or deficiency is not yet known, there are some tantalizing clues.

The history of essential tremor

ET was first reported in 1817 by James Parkinson, who realized it was a different condition from classical Parkinson's disease. The first detailed account of ET was published in 1887, although shaking hands as a movement disorder has probably been around since human records began. Since then, and as scientific approaches have evolved and been perfected, it has become clear that there are a number of quite different so-called 'movement disorders', each of which is manifest in slightly different ways and is caused by different genetic or environmental factor(s). The situation is further complicated because ET is not a simple disorder. The severity of the symptoms varies widely, as does the age of onset, further complicating the clinician's task of diagnosis. A correct and consistent diagnosis is crucial if optimal treatment is to be prescribed—medication that is effective in ET may not be effective for patients with Parkinson's disease, although there is some overlap in their treatments.

The name ET is also evolving. ET was once also called 'benign familial tremor', but the *benign* was dropped (in about 1991) following a study of 753 ET patients in Kansas, USA. A 'Sickness Impact Profile' (SIP) was used to measure the effects of the tremor on patients' ability to perform the functions of their day-to-day life. Using a questionnaire, patients with ET and those unaffected by ET were asked to assess the impact of tremor on their day-to-day activities including communication, work, emotional behaviour, home management, and recreation and pastimes—this gave the investigators a measure of 'sickness-related dysfunction'. A total of 145 patients with Parkinson's disease were also included in the study as a 'positive control'. As expected, Parkinson's patients had the highest dysfunction, but the study concluded that compared with the unaffected people, significant disabilities within all the categories of the SIP could occur in ET patients—ET is not '*benign*'. Similarly, more recent studies have suggested that a fair proportion of people with ET have no history of ET in their family. Although this does not prove that it was not inherited in these individuals, like *benign*, *familial* was also dropped, thus reducing the name of the condition to its bare essentials—ET.

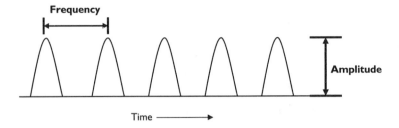

Figure 1.2 Wave frequency versus amplitude (see text). A schematic representation of a regular, oscillating electric pulse as one might find during tremor. The frequency is the time between pulses (1 per s= 1 Hz) and the amplitude defines the strength of the signal (i.e. severity of tremor).

The clinical definition of 'classical essential tremor'

The bilateral postural and kinetic tremor that is so characteristic of ET implies that something is happening regularly—something is oscillating to cause muscles to contract periodically—with a given frequency during voluntary movement. One way of looking at this is to imagine regular pulses of electrical signals as waves generated over time (Fig. 1.2).

The time between the peaks of the waves defines the frequency (literally how frequent) with which the wave is repeating and this, like radio waves etc., is measured in Hertz (Hz). One Hz is one cycle per second. The height of the peaks is a measure of the amplitude (the strength) of the wave.

It is possible to measure electrical activity in muscles as electrical signals are used to initiate and control muscle contraction. The process is called *electromyography* (EMG), which can be roughly translated as the measurement (*graphy*) of electrical activity (*electro*) in muscles (*myo*). Pairs of tiny circular electrodes can be attached to the skin overlying a muscle or several muscles in the arm, and connected to an amplifier to record and amplify any electrical activity arising from the muscle. There is normally no movement-related electrical activity in resting muscle, and it is only when (electrical) signals are sent to the muscle from the brain via the spinal column and peripheral nerves to initiate a movement that electrical activity is detected from the muscle. EMG analyses of ET patients have indeed detected a regular, oscillatory electrical activity arising from the forearm muscles during postural or kinetic tremor (Fig. 1.3) which is not present in unaffected individuals. The frequency of this rhythmic electrical firing varies from person to person, but in ET it is usually somewhere between 4 and 12 Hz.

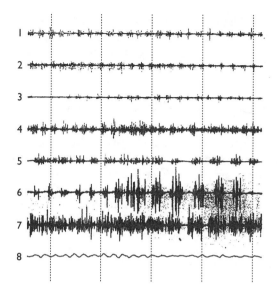

Figure 1.3 EMG recordings. A surface elecromyogram (EMG) recording of tremor from several muscles in a patient's right arm held in front of the body to assess postural tremor. The vertical dotted lines are at 1 s intervals. The EMG traces show small electrical bursts occurring in the muscles interspersed by quiet periods. This is known as segregation of the EMG trace and is typical of tremor. The bursts are electrical signals given out by the muscles when they contract. These rhythmic muscle bursts cause tremor. The picture shows that the following muscles are affected by tremor in this patient: channel 1, deltoid; 2, biceps; 3, triceps; 4, forearm flexor muscles; 5, forearm extensor muscles; 6, first dorsal interosseous muscle of the hand; 7, abductor pollicis brevis muscle of the hand; 8, an accelerometer trace of the tremor occurring in the patient's hand. (An accelerometer is a small piezo-electric device that is attached to the back of the patient's hand with tape. It is commonly used to record tremor and works by measuring the acceleration and deceleration movements of the patient's hand caused by tremor in m/s/s). As the intervals between the dotted line are 1 s, so the number of oscillations within an interval can be directly converted into Hz. These traces are unusual as the tremor in some muscles is 5 Hz (traces 1, 2, 3 and 4), but 3 Hz in others (traces 5, 6 and 7). In a person who does not have tremor there would be no EMG bursts. Instead when the muscles were relaxed there would be no signal and, when holding a sustained posture, a continuous EMG signal would be apparent that is not broken up, i.e. not segregated into bursts. Thus the segregation of the EMG into bursts is the hallmark of abnormal tremor.

Continuing with the wave analogy, the amplitude of the oscillatory signal defines the strength of the signal, and therefore, in the case of ET, how badly one shakes. As will be described in greater detail in Chapter 4, drugs such as propranolol which are used to treat ET have little effect on the frequency of this signal but do reduce the amplitude—the shaking does not stop, but there is a marked effect on the severity of the tremor.

The 4–12 Hz tremor implies 4–12 shakes in an ET arm every second—as the EMG was recorded from the forearm muscles, which move (flex and extend) the wrist, this frequency is the number of oscillations the wrist makes per second. It is important to understand that any one muscle can either contract or relax, so a controlled movement of the wrist requires a pair of muscles to co-ordinate their activities—one muscle will move the wrist in one direction (agonist), whilst a different (opposed/antagonist) muscle is required to bring the wrist back to its original position. The 4–12 Hz bursts of electrical activity that can be detected in ET are only observed during voluntary movement, whereas in Parkinson's disease there is a 4–5 Hz tremor in the muscles even when they are at rest. This is known as a Parkinsonian *rest tremor*.

Essential tremor and emotional stress

The SIP study in 1991 mentioned above also found that although the physical symptoms in ET tend to be less severe than in Parkinson's disease, they cause relatively greater 'psychosocial dysfunction'. One literal translation is that ET patients have greater psychological (*psycho*) problems in public (*social*), and is consistent with the possibility that some of the problems in ET are due to self-consciousness/embarrassment—*anxiety* is another word that approximates to the feelings in ET. It also follows that although Parkinson's disease patients are far more severely physically disabled than those with ET, they are less embarrassed (anxious) by their condition. This raises two important questions. First, is psychosocial dysfunction part of ET or an indirect consequence of having the condition? Secondly, if ET patients could accept their condition and reduce their emotional stress in public, would this help them interact more comfortably with society?

Personality characteristics can be assessed in a number of ways. Most recently, individuals with ET were evaluated using a questionnaire to assess three personality traits, namely:

1. *Harm avoidance*: anxiety prone and loath to take risks.

2. *Novelty seeking*: bad tempered or docile.

3. *Reward dependence*: sentimental or aloof.

ET patients were found to be normal for novelty seeking and reward dependence personality traits, but scored higher on harm avoidance, which describes a person who is pessimistic, fearful, shy, anxious, and easily fatigued.

With the exception of the *easily fatigued* part of that personality trait definition, it is a fair description of what it *feels* like to have ET. The harm avoidance personality trait was associated with the presence of the tremor but not its severity and so is unlikely to be simply associated with tremor-induced disability. What is perhaps highly significant is that three independent studies separated by 14 years (1991 and 2005) and using different questionnaires have come up with very similar results. The other study (2001) confirmed that ET patients tend to suffer from depression and 'psychosocial functioning', but also reported that this was noticed enough to cause disturbance in, or to provoke comments from, the patient's immediate family. These aspects of the ET personality are consistently noticed by the patients themselves and their immediate family, do not require ultrasensitive tests to detect, and thus have important influences on the daily lives of people with ET and their relatives.

Anxiety is a normal response to threatening or dangerous situations that are perceived by the senses. We are all familiar with the unpleasant physical effects brought on by a sudden fright. The response is rapid and uncontrollable (*autonomic*), and involves both neural pathways and the release of stress response hormones, including adrenaline (epinephrine), that are then carried throughout the body in the bloodstream to prepare the body for the emergency. The symptoms of fear and anxiety include sweating, panting, pupil dilation, increased blood pressure, increased heart beat, increased

Patient Perspective

Dry martinis with lots of ice were a favourite family tipple, and these were invariably served with an olive speared on a toothpick. As children, we grew accustomed to the musical sound of rattling ice in glasses, and secretly thought of James Bond who also liked his martinis 'shaken and not stirred'. The process of eating the olive was fascinating as there was a good chance that the olive would fly off before reaching the mouth, and a shaky toothpick anywhere near the eyes is very dangerous. However, the olive was always left to the last, and therefore tackled after the effects of the alcohol had kicked in, thus reducing the potential for accidents. We would never laugh openly (this would be unforgivable) but it was almost impossible not to see or imagine the lighter side. As is so often the case with children, this humour could be quite cruel.

vigilance, increased reflexes, freezing, an open mouth (jaw drops), and unusual visceral feelings such as 'butterflies in the stomach' and a dry mouth.

It is aubiquitous finding that the symptoms of ET worsen during emotional stress, and several of the drugs that are effective in treating ET reduce anxiety and/or dampen the body's response to stress. It is also well established that relaxation techniques such as meditation, yoga and hypnosis can be effective in times of stress. A sense of humour also helps relieve stress considerably. What is not well recognized is the possibility that for people with ET it is the self-conscious embarrassment of the physical tremor itself that causes, or contributes to, that stress in many (public) circumstances—this must be one major reason for the 'sociophobia' which is not specifically addressed by these relaxation techniques, and so they are not particularly effective.

Essential tremor and physiological stress

The tremor in ET also gets worse as a consequence of physiological stress. Physiology is the study of the functions, collectively, of the body. So physiological stress means anything which places a strain on the body's function. For example, it is common knowledge that excessive alcohol consumption induces a physiological stress, as evidenced by the unpleasant hangover that occurs the following morning, when typically ET will be significantly worse. However, physiological stress has other implications. It may be transiently worse after strenuous exercise, but this usually does not last long. Much more difficult to cope with is the physiological stress of hormonal changes during puberty (Chapter 4) or women's menstrual cycle—the signs and symptoms of ET do worsen before menstruation, and the thought of having ET, pre-menstrual tension and a hangover is difficult for a man to imagine. More

Patient Perspective

I first became aware of having a mild form of ET when I was about 8 years old, as physical exercise could cause some shaking. It was at puberty that shaking became quite noticeable, and this was partly due to being self-conscious but I also think it might be related to hormonal changes in the body. However, most of my life I have been convinced that I only have a mild form of ET and so have not let it interfere too much with my life and the things I do in public. I tend to shake when something stressful or unexpected happens, and then it is not only my hands that shake but my whole body and my voice. It is also getting worse with age.

significant, however, is that physiological stress increases with age and is part and parcel of the process of growing old. Perhaps this partly explains why the severity of ET increases with age.

Ageing—essential tremor is a progressive disease, but is it a neurodegenerative disorder?

James Parkinson originally concluded that although there were similarities between Parkinson's disease and ET, they were in fact distinct conditions, separate movement disorders. What ET, Parkinson's, Alzheimer's and Huntington's diseases all have in common is that they all get worse with age—they are progressive. However, the symptoms of these disorders are all quite different. One big difference between the characteristic tremors seen in ET and Parkinson's disease is that the tremor in ET occurs during an action and disappears during rest, whilst that of Parkinson's disease is present at rest and may persist during a posture. Furthermore, in Parkinson's disease, tremor is accompanied by rigidity in the muscles and slowness of movement (*bradykinesia*), as well as unsteadiness. The combination of a rest tremor and rigidity in Parkinson's disease produces *cogwheel rigidity* in which an examiner can feel a cogwheel- (ratchet) like effect when passively flexing and extending a patient's wrist. The impacts of Parkinson's disease on a person's daily activities are more severe than those of ET. Nevertheless, the troublesome effects of ET are predominantly limited to a great extent on movement. In contrast, Alzheimer's disease affects the mind, causing memory loss as well as a progressive decline in personality and intellect. It is now appreciated that Parkinson's disease also produces dementia, but usually after a long period of physical disability. Similarly Huntington's disease usually manifests itself in mid-adult life as involuntary jerky movements of the arms, face, head, legs and torso, but ultimately significant cognitive and personality changes (*dementia*) occur. The progressive nature of these disorders implies that the neurological damage that causes the symptoms increases with ageing.

Jagger and King (1955) made the following remarks about the tremulous descendants of a Great Lakes ship captain who had essential tremor and migrated to Utah in 1860:

'*In two men over 70 years of age, writing, shaving and buttoning clothes were not easy. Of the two, however, one had killed a deer with a rifle at 200 yards the previous autumn*'.

Reproduced with permission of Archives of Internal Medicine 95, 788–793. Copyright © (1995) American Medical Association. All rights reserved.

It is clear that different parts of the brain are being affected in these different disorders. ET involves parts of the brain involved in movement, Alzheimer's disease parts of the brain involved in thought, and Huntington's or Parkinson's diseases a combination of the two. What is most significant is that all these neurological conditions can be very difficult to diagnose, and absolute proof of the diagnoses of Parkinson's disease or Alzheimer's disease is only usually made following a post-mortem and a pathological examination of the brain. Different areas of the brain are damaged in Alzheimer's, Parkinson's and Huntington's diseases. This difference in the location of brain damage and differences in the mechanisms causing that damage, their *neuropathology*, accounts for the different symptoms observed. The progressive nature of Parkinson's, Alzheimer's and Huntington's diseases during ageing is therefore due to the gradual accumulation of nerve cell damage in various parts of the brain over time. Consequently, these diseases are classified as progressive neurodegenerative disorders.

There is no definitive evidence of progressive brain damage in ET. ET brains have been examined superficially over the last 100 years without revealing any consistent or obvious signs of brain damage. However, it is always possible to question the criteria used to diagnose ET in these studies (Chapter 2), and the pathological examinations were relatively superficial because the pathologists did not have modern neuropathological techniques and were not sure what areas of the brain to focus their investigations upon. Nevertheless, brain damage is easily detected at post-mortem in Parkinson's, Huntington's or Alzheimer's diseases, so the absence of any historical reference to clearly visible damage in the brains of people who had ET implies that the damage is very subtle. This absence of detailed neuropathological examinations of the ET brain has not gone unnoticed by the clinicians studying ET. The *Essential Tremor Brain Repository* has been established at Columbia University in New York, USA, so that patients with ET can, after death, allow their brains to be donated to a 'tissue bank'. This allows detailed studies to be carried out and the findings from ET brains compared with each other and with brains donated by people not affected by a neurological disorder. Preliminary results from this approach suggest that a defect in a small number of cells within an area of the brain called the *cerebellum*, which is involved in the control of movement, may be one common denominator in ET brains.

A further major complication in the argument that ET is a neurodegenerative condition is that, unlike Parkinson's, Huntington's or Alzheimer's diseases, ET can affect children and young infants. These very early-onset ET cases occur in infants whose brains are still developing, so it is difficult but not impossible to reconcile this finding with the view that ET is a progressive neurodegeneration.

Even in the more severe and advanced cases of ET, the obvious symptoms are by and large restricted to postural and kinetic tremor affecting the arms, and perhaps also the head, voice, legs and face, without any obvious signs of the cognitive damage such as the memory loss or dementia that occurs in the latter stages of Huntington's, Alzheimer's or Parkinson's diseases. This suggests that either the brain damage in ET is very subtle and restricted to a few highly specialized brain cells (*neurons*) within functionally and anatomically defined region(s) of the brain, or the assumption that a progressive neurodegeneration is the main cause of ET progression is wrong.

Other symptoms in essential tremor

In patients with ET, abnormal electrical and/or biochemical activity has been detected in several key regions of the central nervous system and, in addition to movement control, many of these regions are involved in other neurological processes. Action tremor of the hands and other parts of the body are key features of ET, but an important issue is whether the neurological problems underlying ET cause any other, perhaps more subtle, effects on the body or brain. Furthermore, if this was found to be the case, then would these symptoms worsen during ageing? Many studies have tried to address this issue, but it is sometimes difficult to be absolutely convinced that the neurological problem is actually caused by ET rather than an indirect consequence of living with ET for several decades, or by the normal ageing process. Even if some associated abnormality is discovered, the fact that to date it does not feature in the current diagnostic criteria for ET, or traditional literature of ET, indicates that it is probably very subtle. On the whole, the patients and their families have not noticed it and, if they did, it is of relatively little importance in their day-to-day lives. Nevertheless, it is worth looking for evidence of other neurological problems in ET.

Potential neurological problems can be subdivided into: (1) those involved in mental functions such as cognitive ability, behaviour and personality; and (2) physical problems, for example, affecting walking or the senses.

Cognitive ability

Several studies have examined ET patients looking for evidence of 'cognitive' problems, and concluded that ET patients may have mild impairment of memory, attention, verbal fluency, cognitive flexibility and/or conceptual thinking tasks. This is alarming, but there is some consolation, as ET patients scored higher than unaffected people in several other tests such as 'verbal and non-verbal conceptualization and reasoning'. Furthermore, it is also worth remembering that the anxiety present in ET, the tendency to social reclussivity as well as the effects of treatments and co-existing illnesses, may have influenced the results. The cognitive evaluation studies were carried out within formal environments, with the examiner, a stranger, asking the affected ET individual a number of highly personal questions. If one accepts that ET individuals are inherently self-conscious, fearful and shy, the evaluation itself would have been stressful. This could possibly have affected at least some of the results obtained, for example verbal fluency and attention, so these data are difficult to interpret.

These studies report data for a large number of people, and the deficits tend to be mild in ET patients as a whole, but within that group they range from unnoticeable to severe. Furthermore, any cognitive impairment is always compared with the severe effects observed in other disorders such as Parkinson's disease and Alzheimer's disease, and is consistently found to be comparatively mild. Unlike Parkinson's disease, and Alzheimer's disease in particular, any cognitive deficit (such as memory impairment) in ET is only detectable using a battery of sophisticated and highly sensitive tests. The cognitive abnormalities are therefore of little importance to the patient, their families, the clinician or society, and are defined as *subclinical*—not bad enough to warrant clinical intervention.

Some cognitive decline is inevitable during ageing, so the decline observed in elderly ET patients is not out of the ordinary. At worst, on average, the age-related problems might be manifested slightly earlier in ET than in unaffected controls.

Walking

There is no clinical or anecdotal evidence to suggest that ET tremor has a noticeable effect on movement of the legs during walking. Nevertheless, investigators have turned to complex technology to try and detect abnormalities in the walking (gait) of people with ET. If it is not visible to the naked eye, then infrared cameras, video processors and infrared light-reflective markers attached to different regions of the legs can be exploited to compare all aspects of walking in ET with that of unaffected individuals in fine detail—measured in millimetres and degrees of rotation, etc. Patients walk on a treadmill while cameras follow every movement, and the patients can be asked to walk with their hands swinging freely or held behind their neck, to see whether balance is affected.

In one detailed study, a 'gait disorder' was detected in ET patients, but the defect was only detected in a subgroup of ET patients who had particularly severe tremors and also had '*intention tremor*' in addition to the usual postural and (simple) kinetic tremors. Intention tremor is characterized by an exaggeration of tremor during a visually guided movement towards an object, so that the tremor increases as the hand approaches the target object. It is found in diseases of the cerebellum, an area of the brain situated in the back of the skull that is intimately involved in the control of movements. Intention tremor can be associated with other impairments of co-ordination, for example inaccuracy, so that there is a tendency for the hand to overshoot the target (*dysmetria*). Consequently, in these patients, the diagnosis of ET is debatable, or they represent a severely afflicted subgroup of the condition. The gaits of ET patients with classical postural and simple kinetic tremors were not different from those of unaffected individuals.

As the gait disorder is only noticeable in severely affected people, it may be a consequence of having severe tremor that includes *intention tremor*, rather than indicating the presence of a specific neurological defect in ET. Alternatively, one cannot help wondering whether having a shaking head will affect balance during walking.

Eyesight and eye movement

Poor or defective eyesight is not a symptom that has been associated with ET. If eyesight was a problem, severely affected ET patients would have mentioned it to their doctors, and this would undoubtedly have been reported if there was a significant association between ET and bad eyesight. Nevertheless, eye movement abnormalities have been detected, but again only in severely affected patients who had *intention tremor*, and not in typical ET patients who exhibited postural and simple kinetic tremors without *intention tremor*.

The initiation of eye movements in ET patients with *intention tremor* is significantly slower than normal (in milliseconds), although other eye movements (saccadic and gaze-holding functions) are unaffected.

Sense of smell

The sense of smell can be tested using a 'smell battery' in which patients try to recognize various different odours that are presented to them sequentially on scratch cards, each card coming with five potential answers, of which only one is correct. Using this type of test, a deterioration in the sense of smell is now appreciated to be a consistent early sign of Parkinson's disease. Initial studies also appeared to indicate that patients with ET may have a mildly defective sense of smell. However, recent reports have shown that this is not true and that the sense of smell in people with ET is normal. In fact, patients with inherited ET may actually have a better sense of smell than unaffected individuals. This finding may have important clinical implications because in future it may be possible to use detailed tests of the sense of smell to help distinguish between Parkinson's disease and ET.

Hearing

Deafness in the general population does increase with age, as evidenced by the number of elderly people who rely on hearing aids. If one therefore wants to investigate whether hearing is impaired in ET patients, the majority of whom are elderly, then a number of potential experimental problems arise. One can only determine whether deafness is more or less frequent than expected compared with age-matched controls. One study measured hearing in ET patients, Parkinson's disease patients and healthy individuals using a standard hearing test (*Nursing Home Hearing Handicap Index*). ET patients were found to have an increased hearing disability compared with people with Parkinson's disease and healthy people, and this correlated with tremor severity, age and sex (male). However, this finding needs to be corroborated before too much credence is given to it.

Weight loss

Being underweight has as many health implications as being overweight, and patients with neurodegenerative disorders tend to be thinner than average. For example, in patients with Parkinson's disease, significant weight loss occurs even before the diagnosis is made. The scientific measure of whether an individual is overweight or underweight clearly requires that weight is related to the height (a measure of size) of that individual. The standard measure devised for the purpose of classifying people (normal, fat or thin) is called the 'body mass index' (BMI):

BMI = Weight in kilograms/(Height in metres)^2

Compared with unaffected controls, ET patients are indeed lighter. The average ET patient BMI score of 26 was 5.5 per cent lower than the 27.5 BMI score of unaffected individuals. Although the average BMI score is clearly different, there is a range of BMI scores in each group, and this is expressed as the range above and below ($\pm$) the average which would include 95 per cent of all BMI scores in each group. Thus the range of ET BMI scores is actually 26.0 $\pm$ 4.3 (as high as 30.3 and as low as 21.7), and the control BMI is 27.5 $\pm$ 5.0 (as high as 32.5 and as low as 22.5). There is clearly enormous overlap between the ET and control samples, and a statistical test of the difference between the two showed that it was only of borderline significance.

It is probably not worth overinterpreting these marginal differences, which require confirmation. Even if they are accepted at face value, several obvious explanations for these findings come to mind:

1. ET patients use up energy shaking and trying to control their shakes—energy that would normally be stored in the body as fat. This extra energy expenditure in ET on average represents 5.5 per cent of food intake that is not be stored in the body, resulting in slightly lower weight.

2. ET patients on average drop 5.5 per cent of the food in each meal due to the shaky trip from the plate to the mouth. The average nutritional value of an ET meal is therefore in effect 5.5 per cent smaller than intended.

3. The 'anxiety' present in ET induces an increase in the metabolic rate of the body, which thus consumes more energy, so that there is less spare energy to be stored in the body as fat, etc.

Conclusion

ET causes a tremor that affects the arms and various other parts of the body. This tremor occurs during actions and not whilst resting. It typically occurs when the arms maintain a given posture (postural tremor) and when the arms make a movement (kinetic tremor). In some patients with ET, an intention tremor is also present. This is apparent when the hand makes a purposeful movement towards an object under visual guidance and manifests as an increase in tremor as the hand approaches the object. The self-conscious embarrassment and reluctance to expose the shaking in public (sociophobia and harm avoidance) is increasingly being recognized by patients, families and clinicians as one symptom of ET that can have a significant effect on living and coping with ET.

In the subgroup of ET patients with *intention tremor*, mild abnormalities of gait and eye movements have been detected with sophisticated apparatus. In addition, there is some weak evidence to suggest that there are subtle cognitive changes present in patients with ET. These other symptoms are by and large unnoticed by the affected individuals and their families, and are of no clinical importance.

2 Living and coping with essential tremor

Society makes very few allowances for individuals with shaking hands—hot and cold beverages are still served in delicate cups and saucers or glasses that are impossible to handle on formal occasions. Society does not recognize ET as a physical disability. As a consequence, shaking hands are often viewed with suspicion, as they are associated with alcoholism (delirium tremens), drug addiction, senility or simply 'nervousness' in the minds of those who are unaware of ET. In many cases, the suspicions are voiced—'Why are you so nervous?' or 'What are you nervous about?' are fairly common questions. Of course this increases self-consciousness and makes the tremor worse. It would all be so much simpler and less awkward not to have to explain what ET is, and that sturdy mugs or glasses were available upon request without causing too much trouble or embarrassment.

> *I always eat my peas with honey;*
> *I've done it all my life.*
> *They do taste kind of funny*
> *but it keeps them on my knife.*
>
> *Anon*

As ET is a complex disorder, there are several obvious variables that will determine how difficult it will be to live and cope with ET, and this applies to affected individuals and their unaffected family members.

- Severity
- Response to medication
- Age of onset
- Whether it runs in the family

- Anxiety
- How aware you and people around you are that ET is a real condition, a clinically defined movement disorder
- Diet

In this chapter, we will consider some of these variables, and where possible offer solutions using the experiences of affected individuals and family members. We can first dispense with the more obvious issues—severity, response to medication and diet—before considering the more subtle but more important aspects of the effects of anxiety in ET, and the low profile of ET in society as a whole.

Severity

It is self-evident that the more severe a tremor becomes, the more physically disabling it is. This is a physical handicap and requires greater or lesser support from family and friends accordingly, largely because society as a whole does not make allowances for this type of disability. In most cases, the tremor will cause inconveniences in day-to-day life, but affected individuals learn to cope pretty well at home and, in many cases, require negligible physical support. In more severe cases, day-to-day life is affected, but it is at this point that medication plays its most important supportive role. Nevertheless, family members do act as an interface between the affected individual and society, and this physical support can vary from holding glasses or cups on social/formal occasions, to signing cheques or keying in PINs in shops and banks. Online banking and shopping will reduce the reliance an affected individual has on others, but this requires access to the internet which will be facilitated by the recently designed 'movement disorder' computer mouse and anti-tremor software (Chapter 9). Support from partners, family and friends is often very important in persuading the inherently sociophobic ET individual to venture out into society and, as a consequence, to a greater or lesser extent, they can feel a responsibility to protect the affected individual on these occasions.

Individuals vary in their response to medication, but there are a number of medications on offer that provide alternatives to compensate for this and for the variable severity of the ET. The medication can be taken occasionally to cope with particularly stressful situations, or regularly as appropriate. It is largely up to the individual to decide which is the most suitable medication—they may have to try several—and how often they will take that medication. Deep brain stimulation is the last resort for severely affected individuals who do not respond to the medicines on offer, but this applies to only approximately 1 per cent of all ET patients. Although it is difficult to estimate a number, a large proportion of all ET individuals do not seek medication and have learnt to cope with it.

Response to medication

Nearly all medications (drugs) are potentially toxic, particularly in high doses. The drugs used to treat ET have several effects on the brain, particularly the benzodiazepine class of drugs, for example diazepam (Valium); the barbiturates, namely primidone (Mysoline) and phenobarbitone; and, of course, alcohol. The doses of these drugs often need to be increased over time and can cause drug dependence/addiction (see Chapter 4 for more detail). It is imperative that any medication is used appropriately, which means as infrequently as possible and at the lowest effective dose, to maximize the beneficial (positive) effects on tremor, and minimize the adverse (negative) effects. Propranolol is often the first option because it can be taken intermittently (as required) or regularly. The decision to take medication should not be made lightly and should be carefully guided by a physician expert in treating ET—it is too easy to accept the increasingly popular but mistaken idea of a 'magic pill' that will solve our ills. In ET, the medication is not a cure but helps improve the symptoms and also the disability. Treatment is often life-long and the risk(s) of taking a drug increase with increasing dose and increasing age. It therefore comes down to a balance between how badly ET is affecting the ability to function at home or in society against the adverse effects of taking a particular medication.

General practitioners (family doctors) seldom have the time, expertise or facilities to explore the possibility that the diagnosis of ET in a particular individual is correct, or that medication might not be appropriate for a particular individual. In the early stages of ET, alternative approaches such as counselling are rarely explored. It is often difficult to diagnose ET conclusively outside a specialist movement disorder clinic, so the diagnosis of ET by a non-specialist should be treated with some caution, particularly as a misdiagnosis could have important consequences on treatment, for example delay the correct treatment of the early stages of Parkinson's disease.

Diet—coffee and alcohol

There are two main drugs that are available in the everyday diet that will affect the ET.

Coffee will increase the severity of the tremor, and a straightforward solution is to avoid caffeinated beverages. There is evidence (Chapter 4) that ET patients learn from experience that caffeinated beverages make things worse, and they consciously reduce their caffeine intake. Decaffeinated coffee and soft drinks are a useful alternative, although some could argue that the taste of decaffeinated coffee is not as pleasant as the real thing. Nevertheless, the consensus experience of individuals with ET is that caffeine should be avoided as far as possible, and incidentally this reduces the frequency with which they have to deal with those impossibly delicate cups and saucers.

Patient Perspective

I lost count long ago of the number of times I have refused the offer of a hot beverage in public, whilst at the same time cursing the inventors of china cups and saucers and disposable plastic/polystyrene cups.

Alcohol is the most effective drug to treat the symptoms of ET, but rather curiously only works for about 50 per cent of people with ET (called alcohol responders). Alcohol is widely available and socially acceptable in moderation in some, but not all, circumstances. Initially it does not take much alcohol to reduce the tremor and anxiety in ET so, if moderation could be guaranteed, for some people it could be a real alternative or addition to treatment with conventional medicines. However, experience has shown that in order to suppress the tremor, increasing doses will be required over time. Furthermore, the effects of alcohol in reducing the tremor are transient, and the long-term side-effects potentially very severe, namely alcoholism. Similarly, the following day the short-term effect of excessive alcohol intake is a hangover, and this physiological stress makes the tremor worse. In fact there is often a rebound in the severity of tremor the day after even a moderate intake of alcohol; for example, one or two glasses of wine, or pints of beer. Some affected individuals have therefore consciously made a decision not to take alcohol at all (teetotal), and thus also avoid any possibility of the long-term effects—alcohol dependence or worse. Consequently, in people with mild to moderate ET, alcohol is probably best used sparingly prior to important social occasions, for example weddings. In severe ET that prevents a person from being able to feed him or herself, providing that the tremor is alcohol responsive, taking alcohol prior to the evening meal can be useful as it allows the person the dignity of managing him or herself.

Although it is possible to use alcohol in moderation or only in particularly stressful situations to ameliorate the effects of ET, there are problems associated with this tactic:

- If one is to use alcohol in stressful situations, some situations arise, and others arise at times of the day, when alcohol is neither tolerated by society nor advisable; for example, at work.
- Alcohol will smell on the breath, and this can rouse great suspicion.

An affected individual can learn to ignore the raised eyebrows the smell of alcohol may cause in public if the benefits outweigh society's disapproval and unspoken suspicions. It is enormously more difficult for unaffected partners and family to ignore this reaction if alcohol is used by their partner/relative regularly—however moderately. Whilst they may have a certain sympathy, it is almost impossible for them actively to support the regular use of alcohol, and they can be extremely embarrassed by the knowledge that some people will inevitably suspect alcoholism in their nearest and dearest.

> *Alcohol use in ET . . . 'appeared only too often to have served as an excuse for habits of intemperance'.*
>
> *Critchley, M. Observations in essential (heredofamilial) tremor, Brain, June 1949; **72**, 113–139. With permission from Oxford University Press.*

In spite of Critchley's famous quote, there have been many studies on whether alcoholism is more prevalent in ET individuals than in the general population, but the results of these studies are contradictory and therefore inconclusive. It is not possible to say whether or not ET individuals are on average, or individually, at greater risk of alcohol dependence than anyone else. Nevertheless, the risk is real for everyone who drinks to excess.

Anxiety

Anxiety is a key factor in determining the severity of ET. 'Psychosocial dysfunction', 'sociophobia' and 'harm avoidance' are quantifiable assessments of anxiety, and these measures have revealed solid evidence that anxiety is one of the characteristics of ET. Whilst a tremor may be tolerable in the privacy of a home environment, self-conscious embarrassment in public can make the tremor so bad that it can result in a complete inability to function either socially or professionally. It is this worsening of tremor at just the wrong times that can cause the greatest disability in ET, and is most difficult to cope with.

The anxiety in ET can be reduced by accepting 'sociophobia', by avoiding stressful public situations, treating the anxiety with anti-anxiety drugs, or, by resorting to non-pharmacological (alternative therapy) treatments such as meditation, yoga, and hypnosis. However, the evidence for the alterna-tive therapeutic approaches is weak. This is the sum total of what modern medicine has to offer for anxiety to people with ET. With the exception of the very negative approach of voluntary withdrawal from society, the options on offer on the whole rely on external intervention—taking drugs, visiting a hypnotist, etc. The important question that needs to be addressed is whether a psychological approach can be used to reduce this anxiety in ET as it is very much in the mind.

Patient Perspective

It is disturbing and sad that even after almost 50 years of living with ET, members of my immediate family are still prone to self-conscious anxiety attacks in public. This is neurotic. Our affected and unaffected children are hopefully better informed, more pragmatic and less embarrassed by the symptoms. We have certainly tried to discuss ET more openly and positively than our parents and grandparents, and whenever possible we try to laugh at ourselves in public.

Self-consciousness, fear, embarrassment, etc., are forms of self-imposed stress that creates more stress that further exacerbates the tremor. We would argue that ET individuals may be hypersensitive. However, the mind is intimately and critically involved in defining what an 'emotionally' stressful situation is, so it should be possible to train/persuade the mind that certain situations are not in fact stressful. If the mind ceases to think of a particular situation as stressful, then the initial stress response could be avoided and this would thus have a major impact on the tremor. In very much the same way that tremor in specific manual tasks may be reduced by repetitive 'training' (Chapter 5), repetitive training of the mind may have beneficial effects in ET. Thus, if sociophobia is one of the symptoms of ET, perhaps forcing oneself to be more sociable would provide the repetitive training of the mind required to reduce the perceived stress of social occasions.

Patient Perspective

My grandmother was an excellent shaker, a shaker-par-excellence. Her approach to ET was one of apparent denial. She made no concessions to the tremor and insisted on living a 'normal' lifestyle. This dogged determination to ignore it and carry on regardless is admirable and understandable, and this strategy presumably evolved over time and was the net result of a lifetime of living and coping with uncontrollable hands. One unfortunate consequence of this philosophy was that it was never discussed openly in the family as a whole.

Counselling

Professional counselling should have a greater role in reducing the effects of anxiety in ET. However, the effects of formal public events on increasing anxiety in ET are not the same as those which a typical counsellor would associate with stress or anxiety in the general population. It is the self-conscious embarrassment of the hands shaking in public which causes the anxiety and makes the shaking worse, not the public or social event itself. It is the knowledge that there is a very good chance that tremor will increase so that one's hands may 'let you down' in public that causes both the anxiety and the sociophobic reluctance to venture out into potentially embarrassing public situations—it is 'harm avoidance'.

Any counsellor attempting to help an ET patient will therefore have to tailor the counselling to deal specifically with this tremor–personality trait interaction, and this would require specific training. General anxiety-reducing therapies, such as yoga, relaxation techniques, etc., may have a role, but they do not specifically tackle that one feature of ET. Furthermore, before any such counselling can be considered as routine in the treatment of ET, carefully conducted clinical trials should be performed to assess this approach and provide hard, Class A, evidence in the scientific literature. This would persuade specialists that whilst it is important to treat the physical tremor, it is equally important to treat the emotional effects of that tremor. Once accepted by specialists, this approach would then filter down to the general practitioner.

My hands don't shake—a personal view by Mark Plumb

On the grand scale of life, the universe and everything else, shaking hands do not even register. Compared with other neurological conditions such as Parkinson's, Alzheimer's, and Huntingdon's diseases, ET usually causes relatively mild disability. Apart from jobs that require very fine manual function, for example, performing eye surgery, there are very few other activities and careers that are unrealistic. On the whole, there is absolutely no reason why the tremor should have a significant impact on one's life. If we and society could accept it for what it is, the psychological effects of ET would diminish. However, in many cases, it has not been possible to shake off the wholly unjustified and illogical belief that shaking hands is wrong and unnatural, something that will make others think less of us, and above all else, something we have to hide.

Every affected individual/family will develop their own personal way of living and coping with ET, and what might work for one person may not necessarily work for another as the personal/family circumstances will be different.

A formal dinner party can become a nightmare if soup is served, or if the glasses and cups are delicate and overfull. Whist we can deal with this at home, exposing the shaking hands to an audience is likely to trigger self-conscious embarrassment and stress. If we had the confidence to look the 'audience' in the eye and confidently tell them about ET, without embarrassment, it would make a great deal of difference, even if they have never heard of the condition. People might still look, but that too can, and should be ignored. Professional counselling and support groups would help this aspect of ET, but if you are affected there is a way of helping yourself.

My scientific research career requires the presentation of research results to experts at seminars and conferences. One is understandably worried about the presentation and the response to the data presented, but, if one has ET, one worries about how the tremor will affect the presentation itself. A speaker needs one hand to use the data projector computer mouse, and one hand to point at the data on the screen with a laser pointer. The stronger hand can be used for the more public pointer, but whenever a slide needs to be changed, the index finger of the weaker hand must press the correct projector button once and only once—the slightest tremor in the finger and a slide might be skipped, or the presentation might even go backwards (or out of focus) if the wrong button is pressed by accident. Laser pointers project a small dot of light onto the screen, and the dot of light will move about on the screen with a mind of its own—even unaffected people sometimes resort to two-handed pointing to keep the dot of light steady; with ET it can become a colourful zig-zag. Additional hurdles include the problem of publicly drinking a glass of water during the talk, and having to attach a small microphone to the collar with an impossibly small clip.

I was understandably worried before my first public presentation at a conference. I sat listening to other people's presentations waiting for my turn. The anxiety levels steadily increased. By the time I stood up to walk to the podium I was a nervous wreck—I staggered. Unusually, my voice shook uncontrollably, which is a serious disadvantage in a presentation, and even my head shook. Changing slides and pointing at data on the screen was difficult, verging on the impossible. This of course made me more self-conscious, so things deteriorated rapidly. It was obvious that the audience must have been aware of my problem, so it was not possible to concentrate on what I was saying as all my efforts were focused on trying to control/hide the ET. In those short 15 minutes, I experienced all the full-blown effects of the 'fight or flight' responses to extreme psychological stress.

Afterwards, I concluded that I could not go through another experience like it—it was simply too painful. I either had to stop giving talks in public, a very negative solution which would also add another phobia to my collection (and seriously damage my career), or somehow learn to cope. This left anti-anxiety drugs, or reducing the stress of public speaking. I chose to try the latter first.

Having analysed all those awful ET situations in my life, I realized it could all be reduced to a lack of confidence and a fear of being noticed. This was (and is) illogical and unnecessary. I should concentrate on the message being conveyed rather than worrying about the tremor during the presentation. The audience would probably take little notice of the tremor and, if they did, they would not give it a second thought. It was therefore a question of persuading myself that ET was irrelevant and unworthy of the self-conscious agonies it had caused. I would ignore it and/or forget about it. There was one big and apparently insurmountable problem in the logic: however much I might wish it otherwise, my hands shake!

The only solution that I could come up with was one which defied logic. I had to persuade myself that, as far as I was concerned, my hands did not shake: ET was not a factor in my life; it did not exist. Deep down I could hate it, but in everyday life I would ignore it! I would also respond to the tactless remarks of people who noticed my shaking hands without embarrassment— in many cases thereafter, embarrassment was converted into anger or frustration that I would have to spend the next 5–10 min explaining what ET is. This was my personal way of tackling the 'psycho' in my psychosocial dysfunction.

Surprisingly, this self-deception turned out to be extremely easy. This fairly simple philosophy is not particularly astounding—it is not rocket science. Whilst this philosophy is not 100 per cent effective, it has transformed *my* life.

It can all be reduced to a matter of confidence. *Confidence that ET does not matter.*

Get to know the facts about essential tremor

The ability to deal with ET confidently is very much easier if one is familiar with the basic facts about ET as a recognized movement disorder and that it is the subject of active scientific and clinical research. If necessary, this information can be used to explain ET to the curious with confidence, and there is therefore no reason to be embarrassed. It will help persuade you that ET is just an unfortunate nuisance. Above all, you will also find that you are not alone; there are millions of people out there with ET just like you.

Ignorance about ET is not restricted to the general population. In a 2002 survey of patients who had been living with ET for an average of 24 years and attended a movement disorder clinic, only 24 per cent knew it was often hereditary and only 6 per cent were aware that genetic research had been carried out. These figures, taken from a rather small survey, are likely to underestimate considerably the lack of knowledge pervading ET. Frequently, people live with ET without seeking any medical advice or further information. Perhaps ET may be of no consequence to them, or something they are resigned to living with, but this should not be the case for the younger generation, their children, who have a right to know the facts and what help is available.

Perhaps the most important confidence-building step is to get the tremor properly diagnosed and confirmed by a movement disorder specialist: in most cases this involves a simple visit to a hospital-based clinic. If at least one case has been diagnosed in a family, it is likely that other tremulous members of that family are affected by the same condition, but it is important to remember that this may not always be the case. Furthermore, if you do not have any symptoms yet, this may change as you age (Chapter 3). If ET does run in the family, there is a greater chance that ET will be discussed openly within the family and everybody will be aware of the symptoms, the available treatment, and the chances of a family member getting ET and/or passing it on to their children.

It is much more difficult for an affected individual without a family history of ET to get to know ET without a confirmed diagnosis which, at the very least, provides a name which opens doors to accessing the available information (see Chapter 9).

Early age of onset

The age at which ET is manifested can vary from childhood to old age. There are two peak ages of onset, one between the ages of 10 and 20 years, and the other between 50 and 60 years. The difficulties faced by a child who has shaking hands are very different from those facing adults, who are usually more mature, confident and experienced, and thus better able to cope with the tremor in private and in public. Whilst most adults are tolerant and kind when faced with another person with a disability, children can be very cruel to each other, particularly if there is something unusual in another child that they can pick on.

Childhood psychology is a very complex field, and it is outside our expertise to offer any solutions. Nevertheless, common sense and experience can be applied to the more general practical ways of living with an affected child. One way of preparing a child with ET for the almost inevitable school playground comments is, where possible, to be open about their condition.

Patient Perspective

I was embarrassed by my own hands, embarrassed by my mother's hands, and always acutely conscious that further embarrassment was just moments away. The fact that the tremor was trivial, and that most 'normal' people hardly gave it a moment's thought, was impossible to accept. It was unbearable to be noticed shaking, and if I believed someone had noticed, the effects on my nerves were devastating. The more self-conscious I became, the more my hands shook; the more my hands shook, the more self-conscious I became. The desire to vanish into a dark hole was overwhelming. Self-esteem and self-confidence were instantly demolished, and the whole hideous episode relived in detail again and again over the next days and weeks.

Discuss it; if possible talk about other people in the family who are affected, and try to convince a child that it is an unfortunate medical condition. It is nothing to be embarrassed about; nor does it reflect badly on them as human beings. This may not stop the playground comments, but the knowledge that it is not serious or bizarre will provide some protection. If it becomes a serious problem at school, a quiet word with the teacher(s) might help if they have not already noticed either the tremor or the bullying. Other issues that will inevitably crop up include whether or not to learn a musical instrument, and what career to aim for. So far as playing a musical instrument is concerned, it should perhaps be encouraged rather than discouraged as it will help them both overcome the self-consciousness of having their hands on display, and encourage the use of the hands, which will strengthen through practise and training (see Chapter 6).

Personal Perspective

When you first notice that one of your children has essential tremor, it's difficult to work out quite how badly you feel for him or her. Will it be as debilitating as it is for some, and will s/he struggle as some of his/her relatives do? Will it make him or her more nervous than s/he should be, or make him or her harder and more determined? And, yes, as the years have passed, it has done both of those things.

Counselling may be another possible approach, but it is perhaps unwise to make too much of it in the early stages when the condition is only a minor nuisance. The family is the support group.

Adolescence brings on other ET-associated problems, not least of which is finding a boyfriend or girlfriend. There is no evidence that ET has any effect on the ability to attract a partner, but the lack of confidence which is natural in adolescence may be exacerbated by the tremor. Furthermore, puberty involves enormous hormonal changes which affect emotions and cause 'physiological stress'—both of which can make the tremor worse. Again it is matter of support and confidence-building that comes from knowing what ET is.

Patient Perspective

Acutely aware of how ET affected my brother and mother, I was devastated when I realized that one of my children showed clear signs of ET as a baby. In primary school, she was mocked because she looked like 'a little old lady'. Her hands obviously shook the more conscious she was of them. She also failed a musical audition because her hands 'went', as we say. The occasional use of propranolol has increased her confidence, and she has managed to live with ET and conquer it to some extent better than those of us who didn't manifest signs of ET until our 30s.

Medication for early-onset ET is always available, but the decision to use medication, and how, should be taken carefully, with expert advice.

Raising awareness in society

If one walked into a room full of strangers/acquaintances and announced that one had Parkinson's disease, most people would be at the very least vaguely familiar with the name and symptoms, and take it in their stride. The hosts would undoubtedly offer any help they could, and would make allowances during the dinner or whatever, and the other guests would be polite and helpful if possible. In contrast, if one walked into the same room and announced that one had ET, in the vast majority of cases you would be met with a sea of blank uncomprehending faces. ET is simply not a disorder that most people recognize.

Patient Perspective

I told my dental hygienist that I had ET so not to worry when I couldn't handle the plastic cup to rinse my mouth. She wrote in her notes to the dentist: 'Very nervous'.

Raising awareness is the obvious solution. As affected individuals and/or unaffected family members, carers, and clinicians, we must all collectively raise the profile of ET in society, but need the confidence that comes from being well-informed and supported by solid scientific and clinical evidence. One practical way of doing so is to join one of the charities that represent people with essential tremor (see Chapter 9 for details).

There are many reasons for the low profile of ET in society, including the fact that it is not life-threatening or as serious as some other medical conditions, or perhaps because people with ET tend to be reclusive. However, ET also suffers from a lack of media attention because it is not championed by a celebrity. For example, Parkinson's disease is well known to the public because Muhammed Ali, a boxer and sports personality of the twentieth century, and Michael J. Fox, a famous actor, have the condition and talk openly about it. Michael J. Fox has also campaigned vigorously for stem cell research after he was diagnosed with early-onset Parkinson's in 1991. Internet searches inevitably come up with celebrity-driven web sites which are often highly emotive, but are presumably very effective in raising both the profile and money for research into that particular affliction. It would seem that the pressure brought to bear on politicians by celebrities, and famous Hollywood actors in particular, is difficult to resist.

Although there have been a number of documented celebrities affected by ET, including Katharine Hepburn, Samuel Adams, Magnus Berg, Oliver Cromwell, and Eugene O'Neill, there are no major celebrities currently waving the flag for people with ET and thus it is not in the public eye.

In the absence of a celebrity to help increase awareness of ET, both within the medical field and in society as a whole, it is important that each person with ET or with an interest in ET does their bit to raise its profile.

Repetitive training of the voluntary muscles

In many ET cases, the tremor in the dominant hand is much less severe than in the other hand. This is best illustrated by comparing spirals drawn by the two hands (Fig 2.1) (also see Chapter 3).

To carry out any new and unfamiliar task with the hands, the physical manipulations required to execute that movement must be planned in advance so that the effects of the ET are minimized. Usually this simply involves finding a way of bracing one or both wrists against some solid support and ensuring that all the delicate operations are performed by the dominant hand. What is noticeable is that the success and efficiency with which a particular task is carried out increase significantly with continual practice. If a particular task is not carried out for a week or two, that success and efficiency decline, and further practice is required to regain that skill.

Patient Perspective

My handwriting was never terribly good, but legible. However, with the advent of computers and word-processing, the opportunity (and desire) to write with a pen has all but disappeared. My handwriting is now appalling.

To some degree, practise/training can ameliorate the effects of the essential tremor in particular tasks. Day-to-day existence requires some routine tasks involving manual dexterity—eating, drinking, etc., and specific strategies are adopted accordingly. In the absence of physiological or psychological stress, those routine, familiar and repetitive tasks can be carried out reasonably efficiently.

There is in fact solid scientific evidence that strength training does indeed improve steadiness in ET. One study focused on measuring the ability of persons with ET, and unaffected controls, to exert a steady force with the index finger of their left hand. The left hand was secured to a table and, with the exception of the index finger, the other fingers were bent into a fist. High technology equipment was used to measure movement (miniature accelerometer), electrical signals (EMG) and force (transducer) in the index finger. Increasing weights (0–114 g) were then strapped to the index finger, and people were asked to hold their index finger slightly above horizontal for 1–2 minutes whilst measurements were taken. The things people do for science! What is a maximum load? Why the left hand? Why the index finger? (No broken or strained fingers were reported.)

When asked to perform a constant-force task (keeping the index finger above horizontal under load for 1–2 minutes), the steadiness of the index finger improved significantly in those who completed the heavy load training,

Left hand   Right (dominant) hand

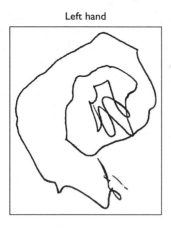 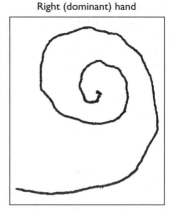

Figure 2.1 Spirographs illustrating the difference in the severity of the essential tremor in the dominant right hand compared with the left hand in the same individual.

but not in those who did little or no training. It is not a question of strength as determined by the power of muscles, although that may play a minor role, but an adaptation in the central or peripheral nervous system, which appears to be able to suppress tremor if allowed sufficient practice/training to either cement the neural pathways required, or avoid the shaky neural pathways, for that particular repetitive task. Unfortunately, the training programme only affected that one particular task and created a superbly steady weight-lifting index finger. The lack of an effect on other tasks is known as 'training specificity'.

These results, which confirm the experiences of many people with ET, are potentially very important. Physiotherapy may help suppress the effect of the ET, but suitable/effective physiotherapy programmes need to be designed so that the 'strength training' improves steadiness in those very specific tasks that are most important in the day-to-day (or professional) life of that individual. The training may have to be custom-designed to meet each individual's requirements, but no doubt there will be some elements that are common to all.

In the case of early-onset ET in childhood, there is the temptation to avoid complicated tasks that require manual dexterity, particularly if the task is in public. Learning to play a musical instrument is one such example, and one that the child may understandably want to avoid, and may even be discouraged by the parents who seek to protect the child. However, one can argue that learning a musical instrument should be encouraged as it would address two ET-related issues. Repetitive training will help control the essential tremor in the hands, and performing in public will help overcome the self-conscious embarrassment of the tremor.

3 The diagnosis of essential tremor

Conclusive diagnoses are important for a number of reasons, including prognosis, optimizing treatment and facilitating research. For example, ET can be treated with primidone, whilst Levodopa is usually effective in Parkinson's disease, and tremor in both conditions can be treated with propranolol or with deep brain stimulation. Nevertheless, a cure has not been found for either of these disorders and, whilst the treatments may be effective in reducing the severity of the symptoms, they do not slow down or halt progression, and can have side-effects. A correct diagnosis of ET is also very important to the affected individual and their family, as it can have a profound impact on how the tremor is perceived within that family. Children can be informed about it—the risks of being affected, the available therapies—but, most importantly, that it is a clinically recognized disorder and not simply some vague nervous disposition.

The exact cause(s) of ET are not known; there are a number of other disorders that have shaking hands as one of the symptoms, and drugs and chemicals can induce similar symptoms. The diagnosis of ET is therefore a process of elimination—some prefer to call it a 'differential diagnosis'—but ultimately, although ET might be the first obvious diagnosis, other causes/disorders are then excluded.

In this chapter, we will review some of the logic underlying this process, and stress the fact that diagnosis is not necessarily simple. In many cases, the diagnosis of ET has to be qualified as some of the symptoms do not fit the 'classical' ET pattern. We will introduce the idea of defining movement disorders according to whether there is too much (*hyperkinetic*) or too little (*hypokinetic*) movement, and how that may be related to brain nerve cell activity that facilitates (*excitatory*) or suppresses (*inhibitory*) movement.

Diagnosis as a process of elimination

The characteristic postural and kinetic tremor in ET only occurs when the brain asks a muscle in the hand or arm to do something specific, whether it is to hold one's arms in front of the body or draw a spiral on a piece of paper. Most importantly, the tremor does not occur when the arm is at rest. The postural and kinetic tremor are therefore readily identified through simple observation of the patient's arms in three actions:

1. Sitting with the patient's arms resting in their lap. This allows a rest tremor to be detected, which would be against a diagnosis of ET and for Parkinsonism.

2. Asking the patient to hold their hands out in front of them, to look for postural tremor, one of the characteristics of ET.

3. Asking the patient to perform the 'finger–nose–finger' test, which assesses their ability to control the movement of a finger to a target. In this case, the patient moves a finger from their nose to the clinician's finger back and forth several times. The tremor present during this type of goal-directed movement tremor is a form of action (kinetic) tremor called intention tremor and will affect the patient's ability to perform manual tasks.

ET patients also have a very characteristic way of writing (which reveals the tremor), so handwriting can be used as supportive evidence of the diagnosis of ET. Parkinson's disease handwriting tends to be very small (*micrographia*) as well as shaky. As handwriting is arguably becoming obsolete and is not always easy to interpret, patients are often asked to draw a spiral on a piece of paper instead—spirography is a writing paradigm. The progression of ET over many years or decades can be revealed by looking at a patient's old letters or writings.

However, this is still not sufficient as other conditions can cause postural and/or intention tremors. Furthermore, ET is so common in the human population that it is not unusual for ET patients, particularly elderly patients, to have another unrelated disorder that complicates the task of diagnosis. The precise neurological damage that specifically causes ET is not known, so brain scans and the like may be able to exclude other disorders, but will not be able to confirm an ET diagnosis. Similarly, the genetic defect(s) that cause(s) ET is not known (Chapter 5), so a genetic test is currently unavailable.

The diagnosis of ET is therefore a matter of first establishing that there is an action tremor, and secondly of excluding, where possible, other causes for the tremor. For example, this includes a careful and detailed history of the recreational or therapeutic drug use (or abuse) by the patient, as many drugs and chemicals can induce similar symptoms. The possibility of accidental or occupational exposure to toxic chemicals known to cause tremors (*tremorogenic*) also has to be considered.

If the postural and kinetic tremor is the only obvious symptom, and there is no history of exposure to drugs or chemicals, the diagnosis is relatively straightforward—*classical* ET. However, if there are other symptoms, for example restless legs or other aspects of the tremor itself that do not fall into the classical definition of the ET tremor, such as tremor at rest as well as during action, then diagnosis becomes much more difficult. When a diagnosis is reached in the more difficult cases, it is often subclassified into 'probable' or 'possible' to indicate the confidence with which that diagnosis has been reached.

To try and standardize this subclassification nomenclature, several schemes have been proposed by a variety of self-appointed groups of movement disorder specialists. There are three main schemes, the first of which was proposed in 1995 by the Tremor Investigation Group (TRIG) convened by the Movement Disorder Society (MDS). The second was proposed by the American National Institutes of Health (NIH) Collaborative Genetic Criteria (1996), indicating that the NIH at the very least is convinced that genetics play a significant role in ET. The third (1997) was the Consensus Statement of the Movement Disorder Society. Overall they are all very similar, with most attention being placed on what to exclude. One such classification scheme that emphasizes the difficulties in diagnosis is as follows.

Classical ET: bilateral postural and kinetic tremor of the hands and forearms, isolated head tremor.

Indeterminate Tremor Syndrome: classical ET but complicated by other symptoms which are 'equivocal' such as unsteady gait, mild dementia, and reduced arm swing.

Possible ET (type I): classical ET symptoms but now have clinical evidence of a second neurological condition, such as Parkinson's disease or restless leg syndrome.

Possible ET (type II): isolated tremors of uncertain relationship to ET. Isolated position-specific or task-specific tremors. Tremors in the voice, tongue, chin or legs.

There are at least two other features of ET that can help diagnosis. In 50 per cent of ET cases, there is a positive family history of ET. A family history on its own is not absolute proof of a genetic cause, but the way ET can be inherited (*dominant*) is consistent with our current understanding of medical genetics (Chapter 4). There are significant differences in the way different nervous disorders are or are not inherited, so genetics can also help include or exclude certain diagnoses. For example, a family history is only observed in 5–10 per cent of Parkinson's disease cases, but as environmental factors can induce Parkinson's disease and could affect members of the same family, fewer than 1 per cent of cases have been confirmed as 'familial'. Similarly, the way Parkinsons's disease runs in some families can be quite different (*recessive*) from that seen in families with ET.

ET has two peak ages of onset, the younger peak being at about the age of 15 years, However, estimating the exact age of onset of a tremor in young infants and children is difficult unless the parent or doctor knows what to look for, or it is noticed (and reported) by teachers. However, in families in which ET has been diagnosed in an adult, the increased awareness of the condition facilitates diagnosis in the immediate family even in infants younger than 3 years old. Such early-onset cases are extremely rare in Parkinsonism and so early age of onset cases in families is supportive evidence of ET in the child and also the parent.

Overall, there is a consistent trend in diagnostic criteria used across the world, but diagnosis is an evolving process as the clinical criteria are refined. However, hopefully, a genetic test should be available in the next 10 years.

Essential tremor versus Parkinson's disease—a differential diagnosis

As described earlier, James Parkinson initially identified ET as a distinct movement disorder in his studies of what is now called Parkinson's disease. The diagnosis of ET therefore first requires that the patient does not have symptoms that are associated with other movement disorders, and the most common disorder that could be mistaken for ET is the early stages of Parkinson's disease. Whilst tremor is a feature of both ET and Parkinson's disease, the way that tremor is manifested (action tremor in ET versus rest and action tremor in Parkinson's disease) and other disorder-specific symptoms (accompanying rigidity and slowness of voluntary movements in Parkinson's disease but not ET) make it possible to distinguish between them. Similarly, ET can usually be distinguished from the dystonic tremor syndromes, in which action tremors also occur, by the presence of sustained muscle spasms causing abnormal postures in the dystonic tremor syndromes. So, for example, a patient with a dystonic tremor syndrome may have an ET-like tremor of the arms, but in addition has a twisting of the neck to one side (a condition known as *spasmodic torticollis*).

Thus the very nature of the tremor can be used to distinguish ET from some movement disorders, for example, Parkinson's disease. In addition, other signs of a disease, for example sustained muscle spasms in dystonic tremor syndromes or rigidity and slowness of movement in Parkinson's disease, can help distinguish them and other movement disorders from ET.

Hypokinetic versus hyperkinetic movement disorders

A 'movement disorder' is clearly an abnormality in movement, and movement disorders can be classified according to whether there is too much movement (*hyperkinetic*) or lack of movement (*hypokinetic*). It is self-evident that a tremor involves too much movement (hyperkinetic), whereas difficulty or lack of movement is characteristic of a hypokinetic disorder. An extreme example of a hypokinetic disorder is the absence of movement in a paralysed limb. Furthermore, the control of voluntary movement involves (among many other parts of the brain) controlling nerve cell activity in an area of the brain called the thalamus which can be either *excitatory* (facilitating or stimulating movement) or *inhibitory* (inhibiting or suppressing movement). The control of normal voluntary movement requires a balance between these opposing nerve cell signals and, when this balance is upset, controlled movement is affected. Too much movement can thus be simply thought of as a result of an excess of excitatory nerve cell activity or a deficit of inhibitory nerve cell activity in the brain. Conversely, lack of movement (hypokinetic) can be the result of an excess of inhibitory nerve cell activity or a deficit of excitatory nerve cell activity.

Although the tremor in Parkinson's disease implies a hyperkinetic disorder, the tremor is only one symptom. Parkinson's disease is actually classified as a *hypokinetic* disorder that is characterized by reduced amplitude and velocity of movement (*bradykinesia*). We also know that many of the symptoms of Parkinson's disease are the result of the degeneration of specific nerve cells in an area of the brain called the basal ganglia (specifically, the *substantia nigra pars compacta*; SNc). It is the loss of these cells that affects the balance of excitatory and inhibitory activity of the thalamus and other regions of the brain including the basal ganglia and brainstem.

The dopamine active transporter scan

The loss of nerve cells in the substantia nigra pars compacta in Parkinson's disease causes their projections to two areas of the brain within the basal ganglia, namely the *putamen* and *caudate*, to decay gradually as the disease progresses. These nerve cells transmit a chemical messenger (neurotransmitter, see Chapter 4) called dopamine, and are thus known as 'dopaminergic' nerve cells. In fact this degeneration begins several years before the symptoms of Parkinson's disease first appear. However, in ET, there is *no* degeneration of these dopaminergic cells.

It would be very helpful if standard brain scans using magnetic resonance imaging (MRI) or computerized tomography (CT) could detect this degeneration of the dopaminergic cells, but alas the scans are not sensitive enough and thus cannot distinguish Parkinson's disease from ET.

Recently, a new form of scanning has been developed, termed a *dopamine transporter* scan (DAT scan). The dopamine transporter controls the release of dopamine from dopaminergic cells and is contained in the membranes that form the surface of these cells. Consequently, if the dopaminergic cells decay or die, the amount of dopamine transporter present within those areas of the brain in which the cells are normally present will gradually decrease.

Dopamine transporter scanning uses a radioactively labelled chemical that is similar to cocaine (*2β-carbomethoxy-3p-[4-iodephenyl]tropane;* [^{123}I]FP-CIT). When injected into a patient's blood, the chemical travels through the blood to the brain where it specifically binds to the dopamine transporter present in the membranes of the dopaminergic cells. The chemical then gives off radioactivity (*photons*), and the strength of the radioactive signal emitted can be detected with a special scanner (*single photon emission computerized tomography,* SPECT). Following an injection of a standard dose of the chemical, the amount of binding to the dopamine transporter will depend on the number of healthy dopaminergic cells present. The more healthy cells present in an area of the brain, the greater the amount of chemical that will be bound to the dopamine transporter. In ET, the number of healthy dopaminergic cells present in the putamen and caudate will be normal, whereas in Parkinson's disease the number of healthy cells in these areas of the brain is decreased. Consequently, the scan is normal in ET and abnormal in Parkinson's disease, where binding and the emitted radioactivity are typically decreased first in the putamen and then in the caudate.

Figure 3.1 shows DAT images obtained from scans of a patient with ET (normal scan) and a patient with Parkinson's disease (abnormal scan with loss of uptake of the tracer in the putamen and caudate).

Is essential tremor a family of related movement disorders?

Several distinct movement disorders can be identified and each disorder further defined and subclassified using increasingly sophisticated techniques. Other than the characteristic postural and kinetic tremor, everything else in ET is highly variable, so the possibility that ET may be more than one disease has to be considered.

'Ultimately, ET might represent a family of diseases rather than a single disease entity. Clinical, genetic and pharmacological heterogeneity suggest that this entity may be a composite of several entities unified by the presence of action tremor.'

Reprinted from The Lancet Neurology, **4**(2), Louis ED Essential Tremor, 100–110. Copyright (2005), with permission from Elsevier.

(A) ET normal   (B) Parkinson's disease

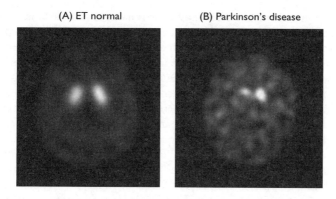

Figure 3.1 Dopamine transporter scan. (A) Sections taken from a normal dopamine transporter (DAT) scan performed on a patient with ET. There is good radioactive uptake in the caudate and putamen areas on both sides of the brain. This resembles two 'comma' shapes, the caudate forming the top and the putamen the bottom of each 'comma'. (B) Sections taken from an abnormal DAT scan performed on a patient with Parkinson's disease. There is loss of radioactive tracer uptake in the putamen on both sides of the brain; as a result, the normal 'comma' shape is lost and replaced by a 'dot'. There is also reduced uptake in the left caudate area, so that the 'dot' is brighter on the right than the left. As a result of the different appearances of the DAT scans, patients with Parkinson's disease can usually be distinguished from those with essential tremor.

The observed heterogeneity of ET could be due to the ever present problem of diagnosis, and that refining the diagnostic criteria would reveal a 'single disease entity' that might perhaps include all 'classical ET' whilst excluding most of the 'possibles' and some of the 'probables'. Alternatively, ET might equally be a family of diseases, all of which have slightly different symptoms/characteristics, but all of which affect a common neurological circuit in the brain that gives the unifying postural and kinetic tremor. The control of voluntary movement by the human central nervous system involves a large number of interconnected regulatory neural circuits and pathways, and very different defects along any one of those pathways could all result in a similar type of tremor, but give different associated symptoms causing the observed heterogeneity.

Current evidence suggests that there will not be a single biological or genetic explanation for all ET—no single mutant gene or faulty group of nerve cells will be shared by all affected individuals. The thalamus may be involved in some cases of ET, but others may have problems in other regions of the brain such as the cerebellum, brainstem, basal ganglia, or cerebral cortex. In all these cases, the same tremor-related neural circuit that connects these regions of the brain may be affected, but at different points in the circuit, and the associated 'symptoms' will vary according to the site and nature of the defect. As a hyperkinetic movement disorder, an excess of excitatory (or deficit in inhibitory) nerve cell activity can be inferred in ET, so it is eminently plausible that there may be a number of different ways to disturb the balance between inhibitory and excitatory nerve cell activity in a neural network. Similarly, as will be discussed in greater depth in Chapter 4, this simple excitatory/inhibitory model is supported by the fact that most of the drugs (and alcohol) used to treat ET act by enhancing inhibitory nerve cell activity in the brain, whereas chemicals that increase excitatory nerve cell activity, such as caffeine, make the essential tremor worse.

Perhaps the most compelling argument in favour of there being several different underlying causes of ET is genetics (see Chapter 5). ET affects millions of people across the globe, and it is highly unlikely that such large numbers of geographically and genetically distinct people carry exactly the same gene mutation. It is therefore more realistic to consider the possibility that there are a large number of different genes that can cause or modify the way ET manifests itself, and this requires multiple targets. Thus, a likely explanation is that when different components involved in a complex neural circuit at any one of several sites in the brain are damaged or defective, they all produce tremor.

There are a number of sites within the neural circuitry where such an inhibitory deficit would have an impact on the circuit as a whole, but all would be responsive to the chemical ET therapies that act generally within the central nervous system by enhancing inhibitory nerve cell activity, or are responsive to surgical intervention that interrupts the tremor-related activity in the neurological circuit (Chapters 5 and 6).

Assessing tremor severity in essential tremor

An individual who has ET knows how badly they shake, and how the shaking is affected in different circumstances, so a numerical measure of the severity of their tremor is of little practical use to them personally. However, a numerical measure of tremor severity is important in clinical decision making and scientific research into ET. For example, the severity of a patient's essential tremor and the disabilities that it causes need to be weighed up against the adverse effects of a potential treatment. Thus a patient with a very mild tremor (scored as 1/10) should be more reluctant to consider potentially dangerous treatment (e.g. deep brain stimulation) than a patient with a more severe tremor (e.g. a grade 6/10 tremor). In a sense this is obvious but, when confounding illnesses are present, for example arthritis or depression, the contribution of tremor to the patient's overall disabilities needs to be carefully assessed. In addition, it is important to document tremor severity in order to assess accurately the effects of novel drugs for treating ET in clinical trials. Most such clinical trials involving patients with ET compare the effects of the new drug with the effects of propranolol and/or a *placebo*, so a numerical measure of tremor severity is required. Similarly, scientific and clinical research requires generally accepted clinical methods of evaluating ET so that scientific data generated in independent investigations in the clinic or laboratory can be compared. The severity of a tremor therefore has to be measured and quantified.

Clinical rating scales

Perhaps the most widely used clinical methods of rating tremor severity of ET are (1) *Archimedes spiral* drawings and (2) using a rating scale to score different tremor components, e.g. scoring *intention* tremor whilst the patient performs the *finger–nose–finger* test and *postural* tremor whilst the patient holds their arms outstretched. However, although these tests are relatively simple to carry out, they are not objective, so the resulting measure of tremor severity relies on the subjective interpretation of a movement disorder examiner. Consequently, in order to obtain satisfactory results with these methods, the 'scorers' need to be trained how to score with these clinical scales. Furthermore, the rater's consistency of scoring can be assessed accurately by using special statistical tests of the reliability of each scorer (intra-rater reliability) and several scorers (inter-rater reliability).

Similarly, there are actually a large number of possible ways to ask a tremulous person to draw an Archimedes spiral to give a measure of tremor severity. The spiral test is supposed to give a quantitative measure of the problems afflicted people have in drawing a spiral, and thus indirectly test handwriting. However, there are several possible ways of drawing spirals, using both dominant and non-dominant hands, including:

- Drawing with and without full arm support.
- Drawing under different conditions that reflect 'effort', i.e. normally, slowly and carefully, softly or rapidly.
- Drawing technique—freehand, tracing a previously drawn spiral or drawing between the lines of two drawn spirals.

Unsupported drawings are consistently rated as worse than supported, and the dominant hand is generally better than the non-dominant hand.

Consequently, in any clinical study, it is important to standardize the way a spiral is drawn before the study begins in order to improve the reliability of the results. To get around this problem, the same groups that agreed on the ET subclassification diagnostic scheme came up with a standardized protocol for assessing tremor severity.

The Essential Tremor Rating Scale

The 'Essential Tremor Rating Scale' (ETRS) was devised so that shaking could be given a number and measured in different parts of the body under different conditions in different laboratories/clinics. ETRS sounds impressive, but in many respects is obvious:

Based on observation and the use of a ruler, a score is first given to a tremor:

0 = no tremor.

1 = slight tremor where movement is less than 0.5 cm in any direction (barely noticeable).

2 = mild tremor with movement between 0.5 and 1 cm (obvious but probably not disabling).

3 = marked tremor (1–2 cm) (probably partially disabling).

4 = severe, coarse and disabling tremor (more than 2 cm).

Patients are also asked to write a sentence, draw spirals (spirography) and straight lines, and perform a water pouring test, and a similar score (0–4) is given where 0 is normal and 4 the most severe.

Writing a sentence:	4—no letter is recognizable.
Drawing a spiral:	4—the figure is not recognizable.
Drawing a straight line between lines:	4—the figure is not recognizable.
Pouring water from one glass into another:	4—most (more than half) of the water is spilt.

Even with this 'standardized type of assessment' there are still issues about what is 'normal' and how the intermediate (1–3) scores are apportioned. Furthermore, several technical details which could make a big difference to the scores are lacking. For example, no details were given in the protocol about the size of the glass of water or how full it should be prior to starting the test.

As these tests may in themselves induce stress and exacerbate ET at the time they are carried out, the patients are also given a questionnaire to assess the effects of the tremor on their *Activities of Daily Living* (ADL).

Furthermore, to get around the problem that any one patient's emotional and physiological stress will vary significantly from day to day, the investigators have to analyse a group of patients and carry out multiple tests on each individual.

Personal Perspective

I have never taken the ETRS test, and have enormous sympathy for those who underwent the test many times during a clinical trial. I suspect that at home my ETRS score would be somewhere between 1 and 2, but would increase to between 3 and 4 when being observed in a clinic.

M.P.

Whilst clinical rating scales such as the ETRS may be rather crude, and the statistical analyses of all the different tests complicated, one must agree that the effects of alcohol or propranolol on tremor severity will be easily detected using the ETRS or a similar type of test. Other signs of severity that are not measured by the ETRS but which are equally obvious to the observer (and patient) are tremor of the head and voice, but these are also quantifiable. Clinical rating schemes such as the ETRS will comfortably measure changes in the severity of a patient's tremor which would significantly influence their disabilities.

It is also possible to measure much more subtle changes in a patient's ET using sophisticated electronic equipment. Accelerometry, computerized tracking tasks, graphic digitizing tablets and EMG can all be used to assess the condition further, but the cost of the equipment and time required to use these physiological techniques make them unsuitable for routine clinical assessments.

The modified finger–nose–finger test

From a clinician's and patient's point of view, the full ETRS test is extremely labour-intensive and time-consuming as it involves videotaped neurological examinations in the clinic. Simpler but equally reliable alternatives are being sought, particularly ones that do not require the patient to attend the clinic. Most people with ET do not attend movement disorder clinics on a regular basis, so the progress of the tremor over time cannot be monitored in any detail. What is required is a do-it-yourself test that can be carried out at home and posted to the clinic for analysis. Understandably this is a subject of active research. Alternative tests are devised and compared with the standard test(s).

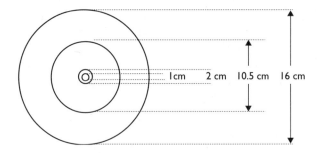

Figure 3.2 Modified finger–nose–finger test target (not to scale). As published by Louis and colleagues (2005). The instructions on using the target and scoring the results are given in the text.

The finger–nose–finger test measures the ability to control the movement of a finger to a target. The severity of the tremor will affect the accuracy with which that target is touched, and experienced observers will also judge the movement of the arm as it travels to the target. E.D. Louis and colleagues designed a modified finger–nose–finger test which can be carried out at home, and the data (two sheets of paper) posted to the clinic for analysis. All that is required is that the subject uses a pen to place a mark as close as possible to the centre of a *Target Practice* sheet (Fig. 3.2). The dimensions of the sheet (not to scale) are given in the figure.

The dimensions of the Target Practice reflect the measurement of tremor severity (in cm) using the ETRS system described above and repeated here for comparison:

Based on observation and the use of a ruler, a score is first given to a tremor:

0 = no tremor. Marks will fall well inside the inner circle. No lines.

1 = slight tremor where movement is less than 0.5 cm in any direction (barely noticeable). Marks unlikely to fall outside the inner 1 cm circle. No lines.

2 = mild tremor with movement between 0.5 and 1 cm. Some marks likely to fall between the inner and outer circles. Some lines.

3 = marked tremor (1–2 cm). Most marks will fall outside the inner circle and some outside the outer circle. Many lines.

4 = severe, coarse and disabling tremor (more than 2 cm). All outside the outer circle with lots of lines.

The modified finger–nose–finger test instructions to the subjects are very specific, and for those who might like to try this at home, the instructions as published are reproduced.

Instructions for marking targets

Materials needed for this exercise:

- 2 Target Practice sheets (attached to these instructions)
- Pen (please use felt tip, because it marks more clearly)
- Tape
- Wall or door (flat, stable vertical surface)

Instructions:

1. Please hold your arm straight out in front of you, at shoulder height. Tape the *right-hand* Target Practice sheet to a wall or a closed door, so that the target in the middle of the sheet is level with your arm held straight out in front of you. *Note: if you are worried about marking your wall or door, feel free to tape a sheet of newspaper on the surface first, then the Target Practice sheet.*

2. Pick up the felt tip pen. Stand one arm's length away from the sheet, then take half a step back (about one foot).

3. Take the cap off the pen and hold the pen in your *right hand*. Raise your arm to shoulder height, lean forward, and aim for the target, making one mark on the paper. Please do not throw the pen or make an X. Just lean forward and try to make a dot on the target.

4. Put your arm back down, resting at your side. Lift your arm back to shoulder height and repeat marking the paper. Repeat this 5 times in total. (There should be 5 attempted marks on the paper.)

5. Repeat this procedure with a new Target Practice sheet and your *left hand*, again for 5 times.

Feasability and validity of a modified finger-nose-finger test. From: Louis, E.D., Applegate, L.M., Borden, S., Moskowitz, C. and Jin, Z. Movement Disorders, Copyright © (2005). Reprinted with permission of Wiley-Liss, Inc., a subsidiary of John Wiley & Sons, Inc.

The scoring system is based on the number of points that fall outside the inner (1 cm) circle—potential score 0–5; or fall outside the outer (2 cm) circle—an additional potential score (0–5); or the number of lines (at least 0.5 cm long) drawn because of the shaking hand (additional score 0–5). Points that land on a circle are scored as if they are inside the circle.

For example, if none of the five points land inside the inner circle, that gives an initial score of 5. If two of these five points also land outside the outer 2 cm circle, an additional two points are added. If any two of the five points result in a line because of the tremor then an additional two points are added to give an overall score of 9.

Thus the worst score for each hand is 15: all five points are outside both the inner 1 cm (+ 5) and outer 2 cm (+ 5) circles, and they are all lines (+ 5). The sum total for both hands is taken and the total score is a measure of tremor severity—0 (no shaking) and 30 (severe tremor). Louis and colleagues compared their modified test with the standard test and demonstrated that they were highly correlated and this was statistically significant. Should anybody try the modified test (mFNF) and wish to convert the mFNF score into the equivalent value for the standard (sFNF) test, a simple mathematical equation will do just that:

sFNF= (0.174 × mFNF score) + 0.743
An mFNF score of 11 thus converts to: sFNF = (0.174 × 11) + 0.743 = 2.66

An example of self-assessment using this test by Mark Plumb

I was obliged to try this out myself—it is not as easy as it looks. My mFNF scores were:

Right hand (dominant):

Two inside the inner circle	0 points
One on the inner circle	0 points
Two outside the inner circle	2 points
None outside the outer circle	0 points
Two lines	2 points
Total right hand	4 points

Left hand:

Two inside the inner circle	0 points
One on the inner circle	0 points
Three outside the inner circle	3 points
One outside the outer circle	1 point
Three lines	3 points
Total left hand	7 points

An overall (unofficial) mFNF score of 11, equivalent to a 2.66 sFNF score. I am not convinced that adding the scores of the left and right hands is valid. Clearly there is a big difference between the two hands but, as has been described in Chapter 2, it is possible to suppress the tremor of the dominant hand through constant use—the relatively unused left hand therefore is perhaps a better reflection of the severity of the ET tremor. Nevertheless, this simple test confirms what I already knew—my tremor is relatively 'mild'.

4 The treatment of essential tremor

The cause(s) of ET are not fully understood, so, by definition, the causes cannot be treated. It is the symptoms—postural/kinetic tremor and anxiety—that are targeted in ET and, in most (if not all) cases, effective treatments have been developed/discovered by accident (trial and error), or by following successes in the treatment of other similar and not so similar neurological disorders (Parkinson's disease, epilepsy, anxiety, chronic pain, etc). Clinical trials, or the personal experiences of patients, provide the evidence that a particular therapy is effective, and whether there are uncomfortable or intolerable side effects. The therapies available ameliorate the symptoms of ET, but the intervention is not risk free—other physiological and psychological processes in the human body will be affected by the therapies. The key question that doctors and patients face every day is: do the benefits of treatment outweigh the risks? If one relatively low risk treatment proves to be ineffective, a more potent but higher risk treatment would then be considered.

ET patients can be subdivided according to the impact of their tremor on their daily lives and their response to a particular therapy: people who do not require medical treatment have no risk; people who occasionally need treatment for high stress situations (low/moderate risk); and those more severe cases where continuous treatment is required, and where risk increases with the potency of the treatment. The occasional use of alcohol, *beta-blockers* (propranolol), *barbiturates* (primidone) or *benzodiazepines* (clonazepam or diazepam) in high stress situations is common, and the potential risk of taking these medications in this way is moderately small.

Continuous treatment will usually start with either propranolol or primidone. If increasing doses of these is ineffective, a combination of the two may be tried. If this still does not provide sufficient benefit, *atenolol, sotalol, gabapentin, topiramate,* and possibly benzodiazepines, will be tried. *Botulinum toxin* treatment is sometimes considered for head or voice tremors. The last resort for patients who have severe tremor and who derive no benefit or have significant side effects from any of these medications is surgery. Two areas of the brain can be targeted by surgeons to alleviate essential tremor, the *thalamus* or the *zona incerta*. Surgeons can then use either a small burn (a lesion) to destroy one of these areas (called a *thalamotomy* if the lesion is made in the thalamus) or chronically stimulate the target area through implanted electrodes that remain in the patient's brain (termed thalamic stimulation if the electrodes are placed in the thalamus). The main risks of this type of surgery in the best hands are a 1/1000 risk of death and a 1/100 risk of a haemorrhage within the brain which may cause a stroke.

Propranolol is the most commonly used medication for ET and is the bench mark of ET treatment. However, it is only partially effective in most cases and has side effects that are intolerable to many people, particularly asthmatics, so many other drugs are being tested as potential treatments for ET. In the last few years, a number of drugs have been tried in ET and include 1-octanol, zonisaide, olanzapine, sodium oxybate, amantadine, levetiracetam, theophylline, acetazolamide and mirtazapine, with varying degrees of efficacy and/or side effects. The data on these drugs are preliminary, so no firm conclusion can yet be drawn about their use for patients with ET. To date, none of the other drugs tested are more effective than propranolol. However, the availability of different medications for treating ET allows for greater flexibility in the clinic, so that options are available for patients who do not respond to or are intolerant of propranolol.

A brief overview of some of these clinically recognized (and other) treatments and their side effects is given below. Understanding how these drugs work at the cellular level might help us understand why they are effective in ET and may thus reveal the underlying neurological problem (cause) in ET. It will become apparent that most of the effective treatments for ET are anti-anxiety drugs which directly or indirectly act to enhance *inhibitory* nerve cell activity. Useful information can also be obtained by comparing the modes of action of those drugs that make the tremor worse (i.e. caffeine) with those that reduce the tremor. In particular, it will become apparent that stimulation of the *inhibitory GABA neurotransmitter* is a major target in ET therapy. An overview of how nerve cells function, and in particular how they use chemical messengers (*neurotransmitters*) to communicate, is therefore first necessary to understand how the drugs that reduce the severity of essential tremor work.

Nerve cells—what are they?

The electrical circuitry that makes up the brain is like the electrical circuitry in a computer which uses a digital binary (0 or 1) language. In other words, a signal is either transmitted or is not transmitted—there is no such thing as

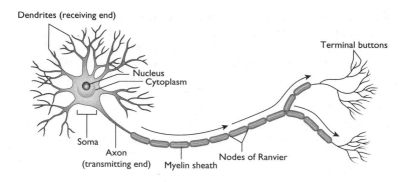

Figure 4.1 Schematic representation of a typical asymmetric nerve cell. The electrical signal in a nerve cell can only travel in one direction, in this case left to right. The nerve cell receives information from other nerve cells at the dendrites, and transmits the electrical pulse along the length of the axon which is insulated with a myelin sheath. The regular gaps in the myelin sheath are the nodes of Ranvier, and are used by the nerve cell to maintain the strength of the electric signal as it travels down the axon. The electrical signal reaches the terminal buttons which connect and transmit the signal to other cells' dendrites (nerves or muscles) across the synapse (Fig. 4.2).

the transmission of a strong or weak signal by a nerve cell (also called a *neuron*). The signal transmitted by a nerve cell is a single very short electrical pulse that travels very rapidly through a network of 'wires' over fairly long distances throughout the central and peripheral nervous systems. The 'wires' (*axons*) are insulated (*myelin sheath*), but connections between cells are required to allow cell–cell communication within the neural circuitry. A schematic representation of a typical neuron reveals a complex asymmetric cell (Fig. 4.1). It is able to receive signals from large numbers of other neurons through a net of *dendrites*, transmits a signal along an axon which is insulated by a myelin sheath, and then branches out into multiple terminal (buttons) which contact multiple other cells (neurons or muscle cells).

Axons, the conducting wires of a neuron are very thin (0.2–20 μm) and come in various lengths according to their function—some can be as long as 3 m. Insulation (the myelin sheath) is provided by support *glial* cells that wrap themselves around the axons to give a 1 mm patch of insulation. The uninsulated intervals between myelin patches are known as *nodes of Ranvier* and are used by the neuron to regenerate the electrical signal as it travels down the axon so the signal does not weaken with distance travelled. The terminal branches of a single axon (terminal buttons) can make contact with, and transmit signals to, up to 1000 other cells. Similarly, any one neuron receives signals from other neurons through the dendrites or directly to the cell body—a spinal motor cell receives about 10 000 contacts from other nerve cells, whereas a *Purkinje* cell in the cerebellum receives up to 150 000 contacts.

The point of contact between the terminal end of the transmitting *presynaptic* nerve cells and the proximal end of the receiving *postsynaptic* cell is called a *synapse* (Fig. 4.2). There is a small gap (*synaptic cleft*; 3.5 nm wide) between the presynaptic cell that is sending the signal and the postsynaptic

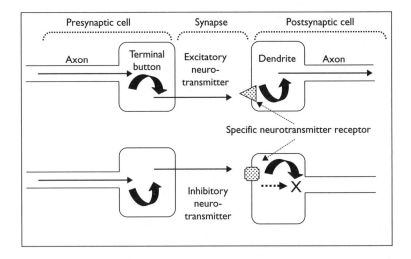

Figure 4.2 The synapse. The nerve cell that that is transmitting the signal from its terminal button is called the presynaptic cell, the cell receiving the signal is called the postsynaptic cell, and the physical gap between them is called a synapse. When the signal reaches the terminal button, the presynaptic cell releases a chemical messenger (neurotransmitter) which diffuses across the gap and binds to specific receptors on the surface of the postsynaptic dendrite. A. Binding of an excitatory neurotransmitter to its receptor (◁) will trigger an electric pulse that will travel down the axon of the postsynaptic cell which will communicate that signal to other cells via its terminal buttons, thus propagating the signal. B. Binding of an inhibitory neurotransmitter to its receptor (▩) will stop the postsynaptic cell from sending a signal. The postsynaptic cell receives excitatory and inhibitory information from hundreds to thousands of other cells, so it is the relative strength of all the excitatory and inhibitory signals that determines whether the postsynaptic cell transmits a signal or not.

cell that is receiving the signal. A chemical messenger, called a neurotransmitter, is released by the presynaptic terminal buttons, crosses the synaptic cleft and activates the dendrite of the postsynaptic cell, thus completing the unidirectional cell–cell communication process.

Nerve cells release only one neurotransmitter from their terminal button, and the neurotransmitter will either trigger an electric signal in the postsynaptic cell (excitatory) or prevent a signal (inhibitory) in the postsynaptic cell. Thus neurotransmitters and the nerve cells that use the neurotransmitter can be classified accordingly:

- **Excitatory** neurotransmitters: including glutamate, dopamine, serotonin, noradrenaline, and acetylcholine (ACh).

- **Inhibitory** neurotransmitters: including glycine, adenosine, and γ-aminobutyric acid (GABA).

The specificity of neurotransmitter action relies on protein molecules (*receptors*) on the dendrite surface of the postsynaptic cell which bind one of the neurotransmitters. There are dopamine receptors which will bind dopamine but not any other neurotransmitter, and GABA receptors which will only bind GABA. As a postsynaptic cell contacts many other nerve cells, it may have receptors for both excitatory and inhibitory neurotransmitters (e.g. dopamine and GABA receptors), so whether or not a signal is triggered in the postsynaptic cell depends on the overall strength of the excitatory signal (dopamine) compared with the inhibitory signal (GABA) it is receiving at any moment in time. As firing is an all-or-nothing process, there is a threshold of excitatory activity below which a signal cannot be triggered in the postsynaptic cell. Similarly, the electrical signal triggered is a very short pulse, so the neurotransmitter must be rapidly removed from the synaptic cleft to prepare for the next signal, and each neurotransmitter is cleared from the synaptic cleft by its own specific clearance mechanism.

The consequences of blocking neurotransmitter activation of its specific receptor can be severe. For example, ACh is the neurotransmitter released by neurons to cause muscle contraction. Released ACh binds and activates ACh receptors on the surface of the muscle and causes muscle fibre contraction. In the absence of that interaction, muscle contraction cannot occur. The toxic effects of *curare*, used by Native South Americans as an arrow poison, are directly attributable to the fact that curare blocks ACh receptors and thus inhibits the action of ACh at the neuromuscular junction—paralysis and death result. Conversely, agents that stimulate neuromuscular communication such as *strychnine* will cause extreme convulsions and a violent death. Drugs that affect the brain (*psychotropic*) by affecting neurotransmitter clearance from the synaptic cleft such as *cocaine* (blocks noradrenaline uptake) and fluoxetine

(*Prozac*; blocks serotonin uptake) also have widespread general effects across the central nervous system.

In summary:

- Nerve cell signals can be either excitatory or inhibitory, and this is determined by the particular neurotransmitter they release to communicate with other nerve cells. Neurotransmitters are thus either *excitatory* (e.g. noradrenaline, glutamate, and dopamine), or *inhibitory* (e.g. GABA, glycine, and adenosine), and act by binding specific receptors on postsynaptic nerve cells.

- Drugs can either suppress or inhibit/block the actions of a neurotransmitter (*antagonists*) or increase/mimic the activity of a neurotransmitter (*agonists*).

Drugs can also increase (*anxiogenic*) or reduce (*anxiolytic*) anxiety. When drugs directly affect brain function (affect the *psyche*), they are known as *psychoactive* or *psychotropic*.

The medications used to treat essential tremor

A 'clinical trial' is the term used for the long and complex process that has to be followed in order to test whether a new experimental drug, or an existing drug (or surgical procedure) that has not been tested on the particular disorder in question, is effective, is not toxic, and is well tolerated. The sole purpose is to gather solid scientific evidence that a drug works, and the data are usually published in the scientific literature having been checked by anonymous specialists (peer-review). Nevertheless, a clinical trial is an experiment on human beings, and the subjects of the experiment are necessarily volunteers who have consented to participate in the study having been given as much information about the risks as possible (informed consent)—this is a legal requirement established after the Nuremberg Trials after the Second World War. There are many moral and ethical issues that have to be addressed before a clinical trial is allowed to go ahead. Whilst every effort is made to minimize the risk, there is a risk, and in many cases subjects have to come off an effective treatment so that they can take the new drug or a placebo (they will not know which they have been given).

Anybody who has an interest in ET therefore owes an enormous debt of gratitude to the many hundreds of volunteers with ET who agreed to take part in the studies aimed at finding effective treatments for ET.

The evidence from carefully conducted clinical trials available to support the use of specific treatments for ET has been classified into the following bands:

Level A: the treatment is effective at reducing the severity of ET.

Level B: the treatment is probably effective at reducing the severity of ET.

Level C: the treatment is possibly effective at reducing the severity of ET.

Level U: there is insufficient evidence to make a recommendation about the treatment for ET.

Beta-blockers

The following beta-blockers have evidence from clinical trials to support their use for treating ET: (1) level A evidence for propranolol and long-acting propranolol; (2) level B evidence for atenolol and sotalol, and; (3) level C evidence for nadolol.

Propranolol is a beta-adrenergic blocker, and adrenergic nerve cells use nor-adrenaline (noradrenaline), which is closely related to adrenaline (epinephrine) produced by the adrenal gland, as a neurotransmitter, and this is blocked or inhibited by beta-blockers. Adrenergic nerve cells are predominantly found in the *sympathetic autonomic nervous system* which is responsible for the involuntary (reflex) regulation of *visceral* function, i.e. heart rate, breathing, digestion, metabolism, body temperature, etc. In other words, it maintains a stable internal physiological environment in response to changing external challenges—physical and emotional stress.

The sympathetic nerves innervate cardiac muscle, blood vessels, smooth muscle, glandular tissues, etc., but are not an integral part of the central nervous system. They are only indirectly connected to the spinal cord, which also receives signals from sensory nerves and the brain. In an emergency, blood loss for example, sympathetic neurons are activated to induce local blood vessel constriction to reduce blood flow (*vasoconstriction*) to the site of injury, but also increase blood pressure and heart rate to compensate for the blood loss and, together with adrenaline in the bloodstream, prepare the individual for the extraordinary physical requirements of 'fight or flight'. Adenosine is an important co-transmitter (*neuromodulator*) in sympathetic neurons, but appears to have the opposite effect (*inhibitory*) to noradrenaline (*excitatory*)—it can prevent further production of noradrenaline and, in that sense, has the same effect as a beta-blocker.

Beta-blockers, and propronalol in particular, are effective in reducing the tremor in ET, but the question is: how? There are a small number of adrenergic neurons in the brain itself, so the effects of propranolol could be either through the *autonomic nervous system* or directly in the brain, or both.

One clue is the problem of getting drugs into the brain. The brain is separated from the blood supply by the 'blood–brain barrier'. Any drug which targets the brain and which is to be taken orally by the patient, must first be absorbed into the blood from the gut, must then travel to the brain in the blood, and then cross the blood–brain barrier into the brain itself. Drugs that target the peripheral nervous system do not face the constraint imposed by the blood–brain barrier. A considerable amount of research has shown that beta-blocking drugs (e.g. propranolol) that can penetrate the blood–brain barrier are more effective at reducing ET than those that cannot, for example atenolol. A characteristic of those beta-blockers that can penetrate the blood–brain barrier is that they are more fat soluble (*lipophilic*) than those that cannot. So, therefore, propranolol is more fat soluble than atenolol. However, both drugs do reduce the severity of ET, which suggests that at least some of the beneficial effects of beta-blockers on ET are peripheral. A likely site for this peripheral action of beta-blockers in ET is on the *autonomic nervous system*. Furthermore, there are two types of peripheral beta-receptors termed type 1 and type 2. Beta-blockers that block both type 1 and 2 beta-receptors are more effective at reducing the severity of ET than more 'selective' beta-blockers that only block the type 1 beta-receptors. However, the neuro-logical defect in ET is most likely to be in the brain, so the therapeutic effect of beta-blockers on ET is complex, with actions on both the central nervous system and the peripheral nervous system

Looking at the action of the peripheral nervous system, which is more readily comprehensible, it is useful to ask: how does the suppression of the *sympathetic autonomic nervous system* by beta-blockers help the tremor in ET? The answer is not known so a little speculation is appropriate.

The *sympathetic autonomic nervous system* responds to emergencies to prepare the body for real or imagined threats. From a biological perspective, *threats*, and this specifically includes fear, can also be defined as physiologi-cal or psychological stress. In extreme situations of fright, even unaffected people will tremble (think of the expressions: 'to tremble with fear' or 'shake like a leaf'), and this is presumably a biochemical by-product of the physio-logical preparation of muscles for 'fight or flight'. One continuing theme of this book is the psychosocial dysfunction (sociophobia and harm avoidance) that is so intimately associated with ET. There is a negative cycle: the worse the ET, the more self-conscious (frightened or anxious) you are; the more frightened or anxious you are the more you shake, which in turn makes you more anxious. This anxiety will stimulate the physiological 'fight or flight' response which exacerbates the tremor. The role of the *amygdala* in ET in controlling emotion (including fear) is described in more detail in Chapter 6, and there is a connection between the processing of emotion in the brain and the *sympathetic* nervous system—probably indirectly through the stimula-tion of adrenaline secretion by the adrenal gland.

Perhaps the emotional (stress) threshold that activates the physiological 'fight or flight' response is much lower in the ET brain—people with ET may be exceptionally sensitive to physiological and psychological stress—and this response thus includes the activation of adrenergic neurons in the *sympathetic autonomic nervous system*. Beta-blockers will dampen the downstream consequences of the brain-mediated activation of the 'flight or fight' response and thus reduce the physiological stress. In part, propranolol in ET may be acting by reducing the cycle of anxiety. Interestingly, propranolol reduces the amplitude (the severity) of the tremor but has little effect on the frequency (number of tremor cycles per second) of the tremor (the same tremor is still there but is just smaller). This provides evidence to suggest that beta-blockers reduce tremor in ET by an indirect mechanism.

Because of their direct effects on the *autonomic nervous system*, beta-blockers are widely used to treat heart disease and hypertension as they will control blood pressure, etc. However, it will come as no surprise that the widespread effects of beta-blockers throughout the *autonomic nervous system* can have side effects. Beta-blockers should not normally be prescribed to a patient with ET if they suffer from asthma or chronic lung disease, peripheral vascular disease, or have a history of heart failure and heart block. Some of the more common side effects of beta-blockers include breathlessness, reduced exercise capacity, heart failure, peripheral circulation problems, fatigue, depression, weight gain, nausea, diarrhoea, rash, and sexual dysfunction

Primidone

Primidone is a barbiturate precursor which is metabolized in the body to give, among other things, phenobarbital. Barbiturates, like benzodiazepines (and gabapentin, topiramate and alcohol, see below), specifically act by increasing the inhibitory effects of GABA (GABA agonist) and thus suppress excitatory nerve cell activity. There is level A evidence for the effectiveness of primidone in the treatment of ET. Primidone was first used as an anti-epileptic treatment and was subsequently observed to reduce the severity of ET. The consistent increase of GABA-related inhibitory activity as the main effect caused by many of the drugs used in ET is no coincidence, nor is it a coincidence that the GABA agonists such as benzodiazepines, barbiturates, alcohol, topiramate and gabapentin (see below) are all effective in reducing anxiety.

Barbiturates are loosely defined as 'hypnotics', so it is not surprising that primidone use has side effects which include sedation, unsteadiness and malaise. However, the main problem with primidone is that about 20 per cent of patients react badly to their first dose, experiencing nausea, vomiting and disequilibrium. This reaction occurs even if a small dose of primidone is taken. The acute reaction often confines the patient to bed and lasts about 48 hours. As a result of this acute reaction, some specialists admit frail or elderly ET patients to hospital for the day, so that they can be observed and looked after whilst the first dose of primidone is administered. In one study, 113 ET patients were enrolled and given two different doses of primidone. Of the original 113 patients, 87 (77 per cent) completed the study. Of those who did not complete the study, 15 dropped out because they experienced undesirable side effects, and five dropped out because they had a poor response to treatment. Primidone had no effect on 4 per cent (5/113) of patients, and 14 per cent (15/113) of patients reacted so badly to primidone they abandoned the study; a 20 per cent failure rate. A failure rate due to side effects as high as one in three (33 per cent) has been reported, and overall only about half of the ET patients treated with primidone both tolerate the drug and show a beneficial reduction in the tremor.

On the other hand, some patients respond very well to primidone, and the beneficial effects of primidone in those patients appear to be long lasting.

Benzodiazepines

The following benzodiazepines have evidence to support their use for treating ET: (1) level B evidence for alprazolam; (2) level C evidence for clonazepam. There is no clinical trial evidence to support the use of diazepam for treating ET.

Benzodiazepines are anti-anxiety agents and muscle relaxants, and include diazepam (Valium), clonazepam (Rivotril), and alprazolam (Xanax). However, studies suggest that alprazolam is probably effective and clonazepam is possibly effective (level C evidence). Benzodiazepines (including Valium and Librium), are GABA agonists. They are GABA agonists as they increase the inhibitory effects of the GABA neurotransmitter in the brain—both GABA and benzodiazepines inhibit the generation of excitatory nerve cell signalling. Thus, increasing *inhibitory* GABA-related nerve cell activity in the brain is one target for ET therapy; there is supportive evidence that ET may be caused by a deficiency in inhibitory neurons or, alternatively, overactive stimulatory neurons. Nevertheless, the powerful anti-anxiety properties of benzodiazepines further implicate anxiety as an important factor in ET. As nerve cells that respond to GABA are present throughout the brain, and include key cells in the brain neuronal circuitry implicated in ET, the effectiveness of benzodiazepines (and the other ET drugs that work through GABA) does not shed further light on the actual causes of ET.

The prolonged use of benzodiazepines runs the risk of both addiction and severe withdrawal symptoms if treatment is suddenly stopped. The use of benzodiazepines and alcohol at the same time is not recommended. The main adverse effects of the benzodiazepine class of drugs include: depression of breathing (i.e. worsening of asthma or chronic lung disease), drowsiness, confusion and unsteadiness (particularly in the elderly), memory difficulties, muscle weakness, and a paradoxical increase in aggression.

Patient Perspective

My mother was affected very badly by ET. She became addicted to valium, and was dependent on alcohol to deal with public situations. As she grew older, she was unable to write without having a stiff drink and only by holding the pen or crayon in a vice-like grip. She drank coffee out of a large heavy mug and when she went shopping she would ask the shop assistant to take the money out of her purse. She avoided any social situations when she was older and was unable to count on others to help her if she needed it.

Gabapentin

There is level B evidence for the effectiveness of gabapentin in ET. Gabapentin is a structural analogue (has a similar chemical structure to) of the inhibitory neurotransmitter GABA and, in addition to its use in ET, is used as an anti-epileptic drug and in the relief of chronic pain. Gabapentin's mode of action is currently somewhat controversial. There are reports that gabapentin does not affect GABA metabolism or GABA-mediated inhibitory activity, although more recent studies suggest that gabapentin specifically acts as an agonist by modulating a particular subset of GABA-responsive nerve cells but not others. Perhaps significantly, it is now recognized that gabapentin also has anti-anxiety properties.

Although gabapentin seems to be reasonably well tolerated, its effectiveness in ET is still at the probable rather than the proven efficacy stage (level B evidence), so that better clinical trials are required. There has also been excess 'pressure' from the pharmaceutical industry to promote gabapentin.

The more common side effects associated with gabapentin include: gastrointestinal effects (nausea, vomiting, dry mouth, diarrhoea and dyspepsia), fatigue, drowsiness, giddiness, unsteadiness, memory disturbances, anxiety, emotional mood swings, abnormal thinking, ankle swelling, visual disturbances, rash, and even tremor. Rarely, gabapentin can cause pancreatitis.

Topiramate

There is level B evidence for the effectiveness of topiramate in ET. Topiramate is a modified sugar molecule that is widely used as an anti-epileptic drug. Topiramate has several effects in the brain but, most significantly, it potentiates (agonist) GABA neuroinhibition and blocks *excitatory* glutamate neurotransmission. Thus, the effectiveness of topiramate in ET can also be traced back to GABA and the inhibition of excitatory nerve cell activity.

An important side effect of topiramate is that it can affect the eye, causing acute myopia with secondary glaucoma. Consequently, it is best practice to have a check ups with an optician prior to starting the drug, and then have check ups annually. If visual symptoms occur, topiramate should be withdrawn and specialist ophthalmological advice should be sought. Other adverse effects of topiramate include: gastrointestinal symptoms (nausea, anorexia, abdominal pain and weight loss), *paraesthesia* (abnormal burning or tickling sensation on the skin), impaired memory and concentration, sleep disturbances and drowsiness, fatigue, headache, mood instability, anxiety, depression, and nervousness. Increased tolerance can be achieved by starting medication on low doses and gradually increasing the dosage over time. Topiramate should not be taken by mothers who are breast feeding an infant.

Botulinum toxin

There is level C evidence for the effectiveness of botulinum toxin for treatment of essential tremor of the arms, head, and voice. Botulinum toxin is one of the most potent poisons known as it will paralyse skeletal muscles and inhibit the function of the parasympathetic nervous system. Botulinum toxins inhibit the release of the excitatory neurotransmitter ACh that is used by nerve cells to communicate with muscle cells, and renders the nerve ends incapable of neurotransmission. In many respects, it has similar effects to *curare*. The clinical effects last for about 2–3 months before the nerves can recover their original function. However, by greatly diluting botulinum toxin, it has become a remarkably safe medical treatment, so much so that it is now used cosmetically to improve wrinkles (Botox treatment). The clinical use of botulinum toxin is restricted to local intramuscular injections to stop abnormal, excessive or inappropriate muscle contractions. It is the unwanted rhythmic muscle contractions that drive tremor in an affected part of the body. So reducing the strength of the contractions reduces the size of the tremor. The main adverse effects are all temporary. Injections into the neck muscles to help head tremor can cause a droopy neck, for a few weeks, if the dose is too strong for that patient. Rarely the toxin can spread to affect the swallowing muscles, so that the patient may have to mash up their food, before swallowing returns to normal, after a few weeks. This problem is more frequent when botulinum toxin is used to improve voice tremor. A few patients experience flu-like symptoms for a day or two after botulinum toxin injections, but again this is rare. Occasionally, leakage of the toxin from the site of injection into the bloodstream causes a more general effect of fatigue or weakness, which again resolves naturally.

Botulinum toxin has been tried in ET, but there is only class C evidence (i.e. it is possibly effective) to support its use. Nevertheless, it is quite widely used to help more severe cases of ET as a treatment for head and voice tremor. Further systematic studies are required to confirm whether or not botulinum toxin is recommended for the routine treatment of ET. Treatment is expensive as the course of injections typically needs to be repeated every 3–4 months because the effects gradually wear off.

Naturally occurring chemicals

The heading of this section is meant to apply to all naturally occurring substances that are widely used in society. Alternative medicine should also be included, but there are no proper studies (clinical trials) on the effectiveness of acupuncture or homeopathy in the treatment of ET. It would be very surprising if traditional Chinese (or other) medicine did not have a treatment for ET, but, if they exist, for the moment they are unreported and thus not widely available. So, in the absence of any documented data on alternative medicines, only three naturally occurring and popular drugs will be considered here.

Alcohol (ethanol)

Alcohol will temporarily improve the tremor in 50 per cent of ET individuals (Fig. 4.3). Typically, 2 units of alcohol will suppress ET for about 4 hours. There is often a rebound worsening of tremor the next morning—this is colloquially known as a hangover. Many people with ET report that over time larger quantities (dose) of alcohol may be required to have the same suppressant effect on the tremor. One advantage of alcohol is that it is (more or less) socially and legally acceptable and is often available at formal occasions, when stress levels can be high. As with all drugs, dosage is the key—a balance between suppressing the tremor and the more obvious and socially unacceptable effects of excessive consumption (this has been discussed in Chapter 2).

Why alcohol is effective in ET is unknown, although the evidence indicates that it acts on the brain rather than on the peripheral nerves and muscles in the limbs. For example, feeding alcohol directly to an arm using a drip has no effect on the ET tremor in that arm. Advanced scanning techniques have shown that the cerebellum, part of the brain located at the back of the skull, is abnormally overactive in people with ET and that this might be involved in causing tremor. It is interesting that alcohol decreases this abnormal excessive activity in individuals with ET, who find that their tremor decreases with alcohol. More recent data have shown that alcohol affects the

Left hand   Right (dominant) hand

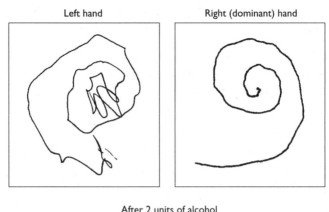

After 2 units of alcohol

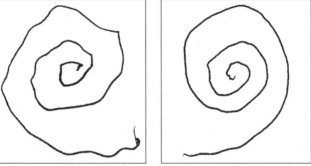

Figure 4.3 The effect of alcohol on the essential tremor in one alcohol-responsive individual. Comparisons of spirographs drawn with the left and right (dominant) hands before and after taking 2 units of alcohol.

neuronal circuitry linking the brainstem, the cerebellum, the thalamus and the cortex.

Alcohol also increases the inhibitory effects of the GABA neurotransmitter in the brain—it is a GABA agonist. GABA inhibits/reduces communication between nerve cells, so alcohol, like GABA, primidone, and benzodiazepines, reduces the transmission of excitatory signals between nerve cells. As aberrant neuronal firing is a feature of the tremor in ET, alcohol may reduce that aberrant firing and thus reduce the tremor. In addition to any direct effect on the tremor itself, one major effect of alcohol is to 'relax' or reduce stress/anxiety—and both may be linked. For example, alcohol causes an increase in GABA release in the amygdala, the part of the brain that has been implicated in the control of emotion and triggers the 'fight or flight' response to danger. It is this 'fight or flight' response in the autonomic nervous system that is targeted by propranolol, so it may be that alcohol acts directly in the amygdala to stop (or reduce) the 'fight or flight' response being triggered in the first place. The anti-anxiety and anti-tremor effects of both propranolol (autonomic nervous system) and ethanol (central nervous system) thus potentially act at different places in the same pathway. Alcohol is addictive, and it has been proposed that its effects on that region of the brain involved in emotion may be one factor in alcohol addiction.

Alcoholism is the obvious potential danger of alcohol use for ET, and a detailed description of the devastating effects of alcoholism is unnecessary here. Nevertheless, a key question is whether the use of alcohol for suppressing ET leads users to the *intemperate* use of alcohol and thus a predisposition to alcoholism.

Investigations in the early 1980s did appear to find a higher incidence of alcoholism in ET patients than in control populations, and up to 60 per cent of ET patients met the criteria for alcoholism. However, subsequent case–control studies have surprisingly found little or no evidence that alcohol consumption and/or alcoholism is any higher on average in ET patients than in the general population. Even so, in some individual cases, ET must be one factor in alcoholism, but on average the risk of alcoholism in ET is no higher than in the general population. Perhaps it is the rebound increase in tremor experienced several hours after excessive alcohol consumption that makes people with ET cautious about excess alcohol consumption, or perhaps, through practice, ET alcohol users have become expert in balancing the minimum dosage required to ameliorate the tremor with the minimum disruptive effect on their own physiological and cognitive abilities.

The effectiveness of alcohol in ET has presented an interesting pharmacological challenge. Any drug that acts in the same way as ethanol but is effective at lower doses and does not have the same intoxicating/addictive properties would be extremely valuable. For example, preliminary data suggest that another alcohol (*1-octanol*; routinely used as a food-flavouring agent) is as effective as ethanol at low doses and does not cause intoxication.

Caffeine

The excitatory effects of caffeine on tremor and the nervous system are well known. Perhaps not surprisingly, a study of 130 ET cases found that, on average, caffeine intake (all caffeinated beverages) in ET cases (138.4 mg per day) was nearly half (56 per cent) that consumed by unaffeted controls (246.6 mg per day). The collective experience of individuals with ET is very strong evidence that reduced caffeine intake is a good thing. However, the 130 patients in the ET study were not specifically asked whether caffeine increased tremor (or it is not reported). The obvious experiment—to determine directly whether coffee increases the 'amplitude' of the tremor in ET using the traditional tests—has not been carried out.

The scientific interest in caffeine's relationship to ET is not simply because of the effects of caffeine on tremor but also because it has been demonstrated that high caffeine intake is associated with a reduced risk of Parkinson's disease. It is therefore important to determine whether lower caffeine intake increases the risk of ET. There is a large body of evidence (genetic, physiological, pathological, neurological, pharmacological, and biochemical) that ET and Parkinson's disease are quite distinct neurological disorders despite some superficial similarities, but the possible beneficial effects of coffee in ET have to be seriously considered. As one of the most widely used *psychoactive* drugs in the world, the effects of caffeine have been studied in great detail and these are worth reviewing in the context of what is known about ET and its treatment.

Caffeine is a non-selective adenosine receptor *antagonist*—it stops adenosine carrying out its function in the nervous system. The role of adenosine as a neuromodulator in β-adrenergic nerves in the *sympathetic autonomous nervous system* and its functional similarities to GABA have already been alluded to (see propranolol, above). As an inhibitory neuromodulator, adenosine can prevent further production of noradrenaline and thus helps modulate/control the widespread physiological effects of the excitatory 'fight or flight' response to stress. Adenosine has its own receptors and, as caffeine blocks those receptors, it prevents adenosine from performing its inhibitory role in β-adrenergic neurons. Within the *sympathetic autonomous nervous system*, both beta-blockers (propranolol), and adenosine and its receptors, play a similar role. Propranolol directly blocks the effects of noradrenaline/epinephrine, whereas adenosine prevents the further production of noradrenaline. Anything that blocks the action of adenosine will therefore block its ability to reduce noradrenaline production and thus prolong and/or exaggerate the excitatory β-adrenergic-mediated 'fight or flight' response. Coffee therefore appears to be having exactly the opposite effect to propranolol and supports the decision based on life's experience by the collective of people with ET to avoid/limit drinking caffeinated beverages. Furthermore, there is experimental evidence in rats and mice that adenosine and its receptors are also involved in anxiety. Anything that blocks adenosine action (antagonists—including caffeine) increases anxiety, whereas anything that promotes adenosine action (agonists) reduces anxiety. This might explain the uneasy (anxious) hypersensitive feeling experienced after drinking too much coffee. Significantly, people that suffer from the very severe 'panic disorder' are hypersensitive to caffeine.

Adenosine receptors are also found in the central nervous system, and caffeine can get across the blood–brain barrier. For example, adenosine promotes sleep as it accumulates when we are awake and decreases during sleep—coffee is often used to stay awake or to help overcome the groggy effects of waking up. The ubiquitous morning cup of coffee to get going acts by inhibiting the sleep-promoting effects of adenosine in the basal forebrain nuclei. However, why is high caffeine intake associated with a reduced risk of Parkinson's disease and may be beneficial, whereas it appears to be a bad thing in ET?

Parkinson's disease is caused by a deficiency of the (excitatory) neurotransmitter dopamine in the brain (*striatum*) caused by the neurodegeneration of the dopamine-releasing neurons. The symptoms of Parkinson's can be alleviated by the oral administration of the dopamine precursor L-DOPA (*L-dihydroxyphenylalanine*) to try and supplement the lack of dopamine. However, despite the development of new and more effective anti-Parkinsonian drugs, the benefits of therapy decrease after about 5 years and side effects are increasingly manifested.

Specific receptors for adenosine (A_{2A}) and dopamine (D_2) are found on the same neurons in the striatum. Like adenosine and noradrenaline in the sympathetic nervous system, the A_{2A} and D_2 receptors have antagonistic (opposite) effects. Blocking the adenosine A_{2A} receptor increases the activity of dopamine and its D_2 receptor, whereas blocking the D_2 receptor increases the activity of adenosine and the A_{2A} receptor. Experiments in animal models of Parkinson's disease have shown that adenosine A_{2A} receptor antagonists (blockers—including caffeine) diminish muscle rigidity and increase the effectiveness of L-DOPA administration in alleviating the symptoms. In contrast, blocking the D_2 receptor induces *catalepsy* (a frozen rigid state). Thus the dopamine deficiency in the Parkinson's animal can be treated by increasing the availability of the excitatory dopamine neurotransmitter (L-DOPA administration) and/or by blocking the inhibitory adenosine receptors and thus increasing the effectiveness of what little dopamine is available. Consistent with this, flumazenil, a drug that is used to reverse the effects of benzodiazepines as it inhibits the GABA system (antagonist), has been shown to be effective in alleviating some of the symptoms of Parkinson's disease. This perhaps explains one of the beneficial effects of caffeine in Parkinson's disease, and has important implications in new therapies for Parkinson's—designer drugs that specifically target and block the A_{2A} receptor. Caffeine, whilst effective in Parkinson's disease, is non-selective and will block all the adenosine receptors and therefore increase the risk of side effects.

A broad general pattern is apparent. Many of the treatments of ET enhance the inhibitory properties of adenosine and GABA, whereas many Parkinson's disease treatments enhance the excitatory properties of dopamine and block the inhibitory properties of GABA and adenosine. At a very crude level, what is good for Parkinson's may be bad for ET, and vice versa. However, there are exceptions, for example propranolol is effective at reducing tremor in both ET and Parkinson's disease.

Cannabis

The West has had a long-standing love–hate relationship with marijuana (*Cannabis sativa*)—governments have tried to stop its use by making it illegal—but the recreational use of this *psychoactive* drug continues more or less unabated. Almost half of all American 18-year-olds (and at least one President) admit to having tried cannabis, and up to 10 per cent are regular users.

The therapeutic potential of cannabis has been catapulted into the limelight as there is 'anecdotal' evidence that cannabis provides relief in patients suffering from a variety of central nervous system diseases including multiple sclerosis (in particular), Parkinson's disease, brain injury, and stroke. Interestingly, the few scientific studies that have been conducted suggest that cannabis has no effect on upper limb *tremor* in multiple sclerosis patients, and has little or no beneficial effect on the symptoms, and in particular the involuntary movements (*dyskinesias*), associated with Parkinson's disease. However, the personal (subjective) experiences of the patients themselves suggest that many of them have experienced beneficial effects of cannabis.

Like many other psychoactive drugs, the psychoactive ingredient in cannabis [THC; $\Delta(9)$-tetrahydrocannabinol] binds to neuronal receptors (*cannabinoid* receptors) which interact with biochemicals produced by the brain as a normal part of brain function (*endocannabinoids*). THC is an agonist, and the nerve cell signalling it induces is mainly inhibitory—it inhibits the release of a variety of neurotransmitters including acetylcholine, L-glutamate, GABA, noradrenaline, and dopamine. The inhibition of noradrenaline release is in many ways equivalent to blocking the binding of noradrenaline to β-adrenergic receptors. The fact that GABA release is also inhibited is of no consequence as noradrenaline itself is inhibited. In so far as the autonomous sympathetic nervous system is concerned, both propranolol (see above) and cannabinoids may dampen the β-adrenergic-mediated 'fight or flight' response. The fact that THC is also inhibiting the release of other excitatory (dopamine and acetylcholine) and inhibitory (GABA) neurotransmitters may explain the many other psychoactive properties of cannabis. However, further research is required to determine whether cannabis has a role in the treatment of ET and other tremors.

As a consequence of the generalized inhibitory effects of THC on the nervous system, the side effects are equally widespread, but additional risks include breaking the law and thus possible legal proceedings and imprisonment. Further research is required as it may be one of the drugs that could be effective, but for different reasons, in ameliorating the symptoms of both ET and Parkinson's disease.

Stereotactic brain surgery—thalamotomy and deep brain stimulation

(1) Level C evidence: deep brain stimulation of the ventralis intermedius (Vim) nucleus of the thalamus (thalamic stimulation) as a treatment for ET. (2) Level B evidence: deep brain stimulation has fewer adverse effects than thalamotomy. (3) Level C evidence: unilateral thalamotomy as a treatment for ET. (4) Level C evidence: bilateral thalamotomy is *not* recommended.

Surgical intervention in ET has been used for over 50 years, and is reserved for those patients who have particularly severe/disabling tremor which does not respond to medication. About 50 per cent of *severely* affected ET patients have medication-resistant symptoms or are intolerant to medication, so that brain surgery is a valuable option for this relatively small proportion of ET individuals. In order to alleviate tremor in a patient's right arm, surgery is performed on the left side of the brain, and vice versa for the left arm. Consequently, in order to alleviate tremor in both arms, surgery is required on both sides of the brain.

All surgery involves risk, and brain surgery is particularly problematical as relatively small errors, of as little as 3 mm or more, can have severe consequences. Consequently, this type of surgery is performed using a co-ordinate system with the probe inserted through a rigid frame attached to the patient's skull for the duration of the operation. This probe is often controlled by a machine (a microdrive) and is not performed 'freehand' by the surgeon. This process is known as *stereotactic* surgery.

For many years, destroying a specific subregion (the *nucleus ventralis intermedius*) of the thalamus (*thalamotomy*) was used, but more recently this has been largely replaced by *deep brain stimulation* (DBS) of the same region of the thalamus using high frequency electrical pulses. Compared with electrical stimulation of the thalamus, which can be controlled by altering the voltage or simply switched off, the surgical lesions involved in thalamotomy are irreversible and carry a higher risk, particularly if operations on both sides of the brain are required. DBS, which was discovered in 1987, is therefore increasingly becoming the surgical treatment of choice.

The target for both thalamotomy and thalamic stimulation in ET has traditionally been the *ventralis intermedius* (Vim) in the thalamus, and the effectiveness of the intervention, and potential side effects, depend absolutely on specifically targeting the Vim whilst avoiding/minimizing damage to any other parts of the thalamus/brain. The accuracy required in ET has been estimated to be in the region of 3 mm within the Vim, with poor tremor control reported for DBS outside that target. More recent studies have suggested that stimulation of another region within the brain, the zona incerta, is also effective in ET and may even be better than stimulating the Vim in certain patients with more proximal tremors (i.e. tremors that are affecting the upper arm and shoulders as well as the forearm).

Evidence from case series performed in many neurosurgical centres suggests that DBS is very effective in reducing tremor in ET, with over 90 per cent of patients reporting marked improvement. In addition to its effects on limb tremor, there is some weak evidence to suggest that DBS can also improve head and voice tremor (evidence level U). Long-term studies have shown that tremor control can be maintained for up to 6 years. The effects of DBS on cognitive, mood state and quality of life (Sickness Impact Profile) have been assessed up to 6 years after DBS and are generally found to be favourable. A significant reduction in anxiety and general improvements in the quality of life are reported. There were only mild effects on cognition, and a small decline in verbal fluency has been found after DBS in some cases.

A 40-year-old man immediately after stereotactic surgery had abolished the tremor in his hands: 'Oh is that it then. I suppose I will have to wait to see if I can hold my glass of beer in the pub'.

P.B

Stereotactic surgical procedures

As the left hemisphere of the brain controls the right side of the body and vice versa, the right thalamus relates to the opposite (left) side of the body. As ET usually involves both arms, bilateral surgery is usually performed in order to decrease tremor on both sides of the patient's body. However, an alternative is for the surgeon first to target the side of the thalamus opposite to the patient's dominant arm. This approach has the advantage of reducing the major risks of surgery by about half. Furthermore, as many daily tasks are performed with the dominant hand alone, the gain in manual function is more than 50 per cent. However, tremor would remain in the patient's non-dominant arm. There is currently insufficient data to make a recommendation about whether the benefit to risk ratio favours unilateral or bilateral thalamic stimulation (evidence level U). However, it is reasonably clear that bilateral thalamotomy should not be performed because it is associated with a marked increase in the risk of side effects compared with unilateral thalamotomy (evidence level C). The main problem with bilateral thalamotomy is worsening of speech,

The objective of the neurosurgeon performing a DBS operation is to pass a thin electrode through a small hole that is drilled through the skull, and guide it through the brain until it reaches the target, which for ET is usually the Vim nucleus in the thalamus. The electrode then delivers *high frequency stimulation* (HFS) to that particular region of the brain. The position of the target has to be determined with great accuracy but, as no two brains are identical, various techniques have been developed to define accurately the three-dimensional co-ordinates of the Vim nucleus within the head of each individual patient. In order to obtain these co-ordinates precisely, the head (and brain) is immobilized in a rigid frame so that target co-ordinates can be mapped out relative to the frame. Different imaging techniques are used to visualize the Vim nucleus, including magenetic resonance imaging (MRI) and computerized tomography (CT) scanning, and in some centres ventriculography (a technique which involves injecting a radio-opaque dye into the patient's ventricles and taking X-rays). Individual stereotactic neurosurgeons have their own preferred and tried and tested method. Furthermore, three-dimensional atlases of the brain have been devised and can be modified by computer programs to 'fit onto' the scanned images of an individual patient's brain prior to surgery to assist the surgeon.

Electrodes that can both record electrical activity of nerves and electrically stimulate the nerves at the end of the electrode are then guided to the target using a small device attached to the frame (a microdrive), or by robot. As the electrode is advanced deeper into the brain towards the target, the surgeon is assisted by a neurophysiologist who records information from the brain cells through the electrode. The cells within different regions of the brain give off different signals, which gives information to the neurophysiologist and thus the surgeon about the exact location of the electrode. For example, as thalamic cells in ET fire with a frequency that is related to the firing of nerves in the shaking ET forearm as detected by EMG, this electrical characteristic is exploited in the surgical aim of locating Vim accurately. The patterns of nerve firing (electrical activity) in different parts of the thalamus in response to passive or active movements of the patient's limbs can further help identify the precise target. Some neurophysiologists prefer to record the electrical properties of the parts of the brain as the probe nears them from the actual electrode that is going to be implanted (macro-electrode recordings) whilst others prefer to use a probe with five microelectrodes (microelectrode recordings).

DBS patients are usually kept awake during surgery so that test stimulations can then be performed to evaluate the effects of stimulation on the tremor and whether it induces any immediate side effects. The electrodes can, if necessary, be moved slightly until the optimal position has been found, in which tremor suppression is obtained with no or minimal side effects at low test voltages. Once the optimal target is identified, the permanent electrode is fixed to the skull with screws, and connected to a battery-powered pulse generator implanted under the collar bone (Fig. 4.4). Long-term stimulation is typically performed with voltages of between 1 and 5 V, at a frequency of between 100 and 180 Hz and with each pulse of electricity having a width of about 60–120 μs. These electrical parameters can be fine-tuned in the follow-up period after surgery using a programmer device that communicates with the stimulator, rather like a mobile phone, in a painless and non-invasive way. In some cases, multiple adjustments to the stimulator may be required. The patient can also be given a hand-held programmer that allows them to turn the stimulator on and off and increase the voltage within limits that are pre-set by their physician. For example, the patient may wish to turn the stimulator off at night in order to prolong the battery life. Typically the batteries in the stimulator last for between 2 and 4 years depending on the exact parameters used for stimulation. The higher the voltages required to suppress a tremor, the shorter the battery life. Replacing the stimulator's pacemaker box is a relatively minor operation. This involves opening the wound in the chest, uncoupling the old pacing box and inserting and coupling up the new pacemaker box. This procedure takes about 20–30 minutes and can be performed under local anaesthetic. It is usually covered with antibiotics to reduce the risk of infection. Occasionally further major surgery is necessary to re-position electrodes that are suboptimal, or have become displaced. At the end of the day, it is worth noting that a foreign object has been lodged in the brain, and it is immobilized by screws in the skull, so there is a small but real risk of infection occurring around the implanted components, or that the body will mount an immune/inflammatory response against that object. Nevertheless, women have had successful pregnancies with implanted DBS systems.

(A)

(B)

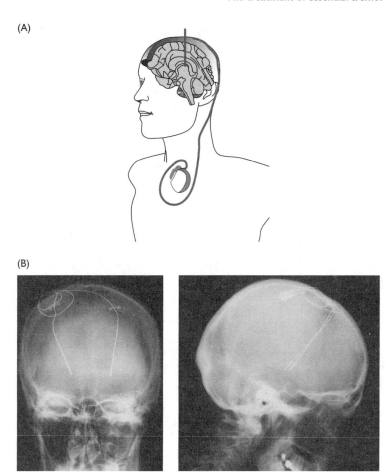

Figure 4.4 DBS electrode implantation. (A) Schematic representation of the DBS electrode in the thalmus that has been bolted in place to the surface of the skull (for true scale; see B), with the power supply implanted under the collar bone. The control of the power supply is regulated using a remote control. (B) X-rays of the implanted electrodes in the brain and exiting leads.

Surgical complications

The main risk of DBS or thalamotomy is a haemorrhage within the skull caused by the electrode damaging a blood vessel whilst being pushed through the brain towards the thalamus. If the haemorrhage is small, minor symptoms, or at worst a stroke, might occur. The latter might resolve over the course of a few months or produce permanent deficits such as weakness, or paralysis or numbness in the contralateral limbs, or speech impairment. However, if a major haemorrhage develops, then death may occur. Even in the most capable hands, the risk of an intracerebral haemorrhage is approximately 1 per cent irrespective of whether a thalamic DBS or thalamotomy is performed, and the risk of death is about 1/1000. A further potential complication of stereotactic surgery is epilepsy, although this is rare and can usually be controlled with medication.

If one also includes the numerous adjustments required shortly after surgery to optimize the stimulation parameters to maximize tremor relief and minimize side effects, the whole process of DBS is very labour intensive, can last for a lifetime and, as a consequence, is very expensive. However, by reducing the patient's handicap and dependence on support as well as need for medications, there may also be some economic advantages.

> *In follow-up [of 81 DBS patients], 2.5% had infections requiring system removal, 3.7% had infections requiring implantable pulse generator (IPG) removal, 12.5% had misplaced leads, and 26.2% had hardware complications including lead migration, lead fracture, extension erosion, extension fracture, and IPG malfunction.*
>
> *Lyons, K.E., Wilkinson, S.B., Overman, J. and Pahwa, R. Surgical hardware complications of subthalmic stimulation: a series of 160 procedures, Neurology, 63, 612–616 (2004). Reprinted with permission from Lippincott, Williams and Wilkins.*

The psychological effects of multiple hospital visits, the prospects of repeat surgery and/or the side effects (however reversible), etc. on the psychological well-being of the patient have not been well documented. Perhaps the long-term benefits of DBS outweigh all the other short-term inconveniences, but some psychological stress in the DBS procedure is inevitable. Furthermore, the social adaption required by a person with ET and their family after surgery is quite significant, as the patient may be expected to perform many everyday tasks that they have not done for years. This expectation and its effect on the patient can produce social conflicts within the family.

Side effects

Some of the side effects can be reversed by adjusting the stimulator's settings (parameters). The clinical names and an explanation of these adverse effects are:

- *Paraesthesia*: abnormal sensation on the surface of the body. With DBS this is usually a tingling sensation.

- *Dysarthria*: difficulty speaking or slurred speech.
- *Hemiparesis*: weakness down one side of the body, typically affecting one half of the face, arm and leg.
- *Dystonia*: sustained abnormal postures and slow writhing movements, due in part to the simultaneous contraction (co-contraction) of agonist and antagonist muscles.

How does DBS work?

As is so often the case in ET, the short answer is that we do not really know, but it is the subject of active research both in humans and animals, including rats and monkeys. There are a few clues to the mechanism of DBS.

Although thalamotomy is now less frequently performed, there is no question that the irreversible destruction of brain cells in thalamotomy can have the same effect on tremor as DBS. This immediately suggests that whatever the precise mechanism, DBS is inhibiting the function of the same nerve cells as those that are destroyed in thalamotomy. However, the observation that DBS increases blood supply to the brain cortex suggests that whilst DBS and thalamatomy may have the same overall effect on tremor, the mechanism(s) may be quite different.

The role of GABA as one of the main inhibitory neurotransmitters in the brain has already been described, and there is one report suggesting that the injection of a GABA agonist (*muscimol*) directly into the Vim nucleus of the thalamus (carried out during surgery for DBS) is just as effective in reducing tremor as electrical stimulation. However, pharmacological treatments of ET do not alter the frequency of the tremor, but are effective because they reduce the amplitude (severity) of the tremor. In contrast, DBS has significant effects on the tremor-related electrical activity of the neurons in the thalamus that fire with the same frequency as the tremor in the patient's arms detected by EMG. Thus DBS reduces the amplitude (severity), increases the frequency but decreases the regularity of the hand tremor. However, whilst this may be true for individual nerve cells, it also applies to collections of interconnected nerve cells within the thalamus. It is therefore perhaps more accurate to describe the effects of high frequency stimulation in DBS as 'inhibiting' the function of a region of the thalamus as a whole rather than inhibiting a specific subset of nerve cells.

One very plausible model to explain how DBS works is 'jamming'. Military communications and other systems (e.g. radar) that rely on radio waves can be 'jammed' by broadcasting 'white noise' at the same frequency, and this has been widely exploited to confound the communications system(s) of the enemy. As tremor is the result of abnormal electrical communications between nerve cells, the fact that this communication can be interrupted by high frequency stimulation makes the word 'jamming' most appropriate. During voluntary movement in ET, feedback loops from the muscles and cortex result in the (abnormal) periodic firing of nerve cells in the Vim nucleus, resulting in regular (4–12 Hz) electrical spikes that lead eventually to the (postural/kinetic) tremor in the muscles. It may be that high frequency stimulation fills the gap between these regular electrical bursts from the Vim, and therefore the outgoing electrical signal no longer has the regular oscillating frequency that leads to tremor. Unlike pharmacological interventions which decrease the amplitude but not the frequency of the tremor, DBS will therefore fundamentally change the properties of the tremor-associated electrical bursts (amplitude and frequency).

DBS may either jam a circuit, or may have a very specific local effect on the site (Vim) of stimulation. There is evidence that DBS does transiently shut down all nerve cell firing (both excitatory and inhibitory), but the precise mechanism(s) that produce the clinical benefits of DBS in ET are poorly understood. There is no doubt that high frequency stimulation does have direct effects on the biochemistry within individual (and collections of) nerve cells in addition to the 'jamming' hypothesis described. Nevertheless, the jamming hypothesis is largely consistent with the data available.

5   Who gets essential tremor?

One of the main characteristics of ET is that it often runs in families—it is inherited, hence its original description as 'familial essential tremor'. In these cases, there is a defective *gene* (gene *mutation*) in the family and ET is *highly heritable*. However, there are affected individuals with no obvious family history, so the 'familial' was dropped. Gen*ET*ics can predict the probability that a child will be affected in an affected family as it is inherited as a *dominant genetic trait*, but in the absence of a family history it is currently not possible to predict who else is at risk of getting ET.

The technical word for affected individuals with no family history is '*sporadic*'—it occurs infrequently and at irregular intervals. The causes of sporadic ET are unknown, but there are three obvious possibilities:

1. It is caused by exposure to neurotoxic chemicals in the environment or diet.

2. The absence of a family history does not necessarily mean it is not inherited. Some cases of ET may be inherited as a *recessive genetic trait*, but this is much more difficult to trace in a family.

3. Some sporadic ET cases could have arisen by a new *genetic mutation* in the sperm or egg of one of their unaffected parents, or early in the affected individual's development in the womb after conception—this is called a *de novo* (new) gene mutation. It is a matter of chance (bad luck), and the ET may or may not be passed on to future generations depending on whether the *de novo* gene mutation is present in the *germline* (eggs or sperm of the affected individual).

The possibility that environmental pollutants may cause ET has enormous implications and is a major concern. Regrettably, there is currently no solid evidence for environmental factors as causal in ET so, if they exist, we do not know how to avoid them. Levels of lead and other heavy metals in the blood have been analysed in ET patients as heavy metals are recognized tremorogenic neurotoxic chemicals, but the results are inconclusive.

Environmental factors are the subject of ongoing active research, but for the moment there is little more that can be added to this potentially very important issue, except to remind ourselves that in science, 'the absence of evidence is not evidence of absence'.

To return to the 'Who gets essential tremor?' title of this chapter, the only answer currently available is in gen*ET*ics which we will go on to cover in a little more detail as it can be used to predict the chances of being affected or of having an affected child if it does run in the family. Moreover, medical genetics is also being exploited to identify the genes and gene mutations that cause inherited disorders, and this is of enormous value in trying to understand the fundamental biological defects that cause the disorder. We will therefore also review current progress in the identification of some of the ET-causing genes (*ETM1* and *ETM2*), but will stress that there are many others yet to be discovered.

Perhaps an equally important point is first to emphasize that it is an extremely common movement disorder—there are millions of other affected individuals across the globe. Some may find this reassuring—you are not alone.

The prevalence of essential tremor in the general population

ET is the most common 'movement disorder' in the world. Current estimates suggest it affects between 40 and 400 people in every 10 000 (between 0.4 and 4 per cent of all human beings). The estimates vary by an order of magnitude (10-fold) and are highly inaccurate, but there are several reasons why a more precise number cannot be given.

1. It is not possible to carry out a door to door survey in a neighbourhood chosen at random to try and obtain an estimate of the proportion of people in that population that have shaking hands—a proper diagnosis is required.

2. General practitioners can estimate the proportion of their patients that come through their practice for any reason with shaking hands. However, unless ET was properly diagnosed, it is also a crude estimate.

3. Many people with ET seldom if ever have their ET diagnosed by a movement disorder specialist, and the proportion of unreported or unrecognized cases varies enormously from one geographic region to another.

4. There may be different prevalences of ET in different populations.

The best estimate for the incidence of ET in the general population is in the region of 1 in 100 people (1 per cent). In comparison, roughly 13 in

100 000 (0.013 per cent) people are affected by Parkinson's disease. The 1 per cent incidence of ET in the general population is striking—the number of people affected by ET worldwide is huge—over half a million people in the UK and perhaps 10 million in the USA. Even if the 1 per cent estimate is an approximation, ET is clearly very common and this explains why the medical and scientific communities take it so seriously. For example, a total of 1187 scientific research papers have been published on ET since 1960, and there has been a sharp increase in the publication rate over the last 10 years.

Men and women are equally likely to have ET (it is not sex-linked), and although the average age at which the symptoms appear is middle age (mean age of onset is 45 years old), the tremor is detectable in about 50 per cent of cases before 15 years of age (early onset). Again this is a crude estimate. However, it is reported that women are six times more likely to develop head tremor than men, but preliminary data suggest that early-onset ET is 2.5 times more likely in males than females, so gender can affect the progression of ET. The symptoms can arise during childhood or adolescence and then be intermittent or disappear for many years before re-emerging in middle age. Similarly, the symptoms do not always get worse with age; although this is usually the case, this can vary significantly between individuals even within the same family, all of which underlines the inherent complexity of ET.

Estimates of the proportion of affected individuals with a family history of ET vary from 20 to 90 per cent, and again this may be partly due to difficulties in diagnosis as the symptoms and signs of ET may not be conclusive in other family members, particularly the younger ones. The best estimate is probably that somewhere in the region of 50 per cent of ET cases have other affected close relatives. However, the absence of a family history does not necessarily mean that it was not inherited, or that environmental factors are not responsible. One other possibility which has to be considered is that in some cases both genetics and environmental factors might cause ET—neither on its own is sufficient, but it is the interaction between the environment and the genes that causes ET. Inheritance might predispose an individual to the adverse effects of the environment.

Essential tremor in families

GenETics is currently the only convincing known cause for ET. GenETics can be defined as the study of inherited traits. In most cases, such as eye and hair colour or ET, this trait is visible—this is known as a *phenotype* (appearance). The unit of inheritance is a *gene* which is a length of DNA (deoxyribonucleic acid) that encodes a protein, and it is the protein that causes or contributes to the observed phenotype. The information to make a protein in the DNA is encoded by four bases which are commonly known by the letters A, T, G and C, and human DNA is composed of a 3 000 000 000 base long sequence of the four letters, encodes 25 000–30 000 genes, and is split into 23 manageable chunks of DNA called *chromosomes* (chromosomes 1–22, and X or Y). A protein is thus encoded in a gene by the precise sequence of the four letters, and a change to that four-letter DNA sequence in a gene can affect the function of the encoded protein and thus potentially give a phenotype. There are enormous numbers of DNA sequence changes in each and every gene in the human population, and these differences give rise to slight changes in protein function that have no significant effects on health, so that, with the exception of identical twins, no two individuals are genetically identical. This genetic diversity is one reason why we are all phenotypically unique—we all look different from each other.

Medical genetics has been widely used to identify and characterize the precise changes in gene DNA sequences that give rise to inherited human disorders such as early-onset Parkinson's disease (Parkin gene), a common form of mental retardation in boys known as the fragile X syndrome (FMR1 gene) and Huntington's disease (HD gene), to name but a few. Because these gene sequence changes have such severe consequences for human health, they are called 'mutations' or 'genetic defects'. However, gene mutations can also be beneficial and improve the function of the protein encoded. If this beneficial change gives the individual a small advantage in the ability to pass that gene on to their children compared with other individuals in the general population, then, over many generations, the number of people that carry the mutant gene will gradually increase. In contrast, gene mutations that prevent or reduce an individual's ability to have children are relatively rare as they confer a selective disadvantage and are less likely to be passed on to future generations. This is Darwin's theory of evolution (natural selection and survival of the fittest) interpreted at the molecular level of a gene. Because ET is so common in the general population, on average, the genetic defect(s) that cause ET cannot affect the ability to find a partner, have children and pass on the defective gene. In fact it has been suggested that people with ET are more fertile, have more children and live longer than unaffected people.

Essential tremor as a dominant genetic trait

We all inherited one copy of each gene from our mother and one copy from our father—most of our cells carry two copies of each chromosome and these cells are known as *diploid* (two copies). When we have a child, we will only pass on one of the two copies of each of the 25 000–30 000 genes in one set of each of the 23 chromosomes in a sperm and egg which each have one copy (they are *haploid*)—most of the cells in the child will thus be *diploid*. However, whether we pass on the gene that we inherited from our mother or from our father is a matter of chance—there is a 1 in 2 (50 per cent) chance that one or the other gene or chromosome is passed on through an egg or sperm.

In terms of a gene mutation that causes a phenotype, the inheritance of a single defective gene does not necessarily mean that the individual will be affected as they will have inherited a normal gene from the other parent, and the presence of the normal gene can be sufficient to prevent the phenotype. This is known as a *recessive* genetic trait. Both copies of the gene have to be mutated to show a phenotype, and carriers who have only one mutant gene are unaffected. When the inheritance of only one mutated gene is sufficient to give the phenotype, the other copy can be normal but is not sufficient to prevent the phenotype—this is called a *dominant* genetic trait.

The way a trait is inherited in large families over several generations allows geneticists to distinguish between dominant and recessive genetic traits, and this can be summarized as follows:

- In a dominant inherited trait, an affected individual will have at least one affected parent. In large families, affected individuals will be found in every generation.

- In a recessive trait, there may be no family history as parents and/or grandparents were carriers and were therefore not affected. Where a family history can be found, it is not unusual for recessive traits to skip generation(s).

ET is a dominant inherited trait but, before looking at the way ET is inherited, it is worth first looking at inheritance in a typical recessive inherited trait for comparison. We will use sickle cell anaemia as an example.

Sickle cell anaemia is a recessive genetic disorder and is caused by a mutation in the β-globin gene. The normal β-globin gene is called β-A_1 and the mutant globin gene is called β-S. Affected people will have inherited two copies of the β-S gene (β-S/β-S), unaffected carriers will have inherited a normal gene and a mutant gene (β-S/β-A_1; *sickle cell trait*), and all other individuals will have two normal copies (β-A_1/β-A_1). In most cases, the parents of affected individuals were unaffected β-A_1/β-S carriers, and each parent has a 50 per cent chance of passing on the β-A_1 or β-S genes to their children. As the child has to inherit the β-S genes from both mother (50 per cent chance) and father (50 per cent chance), on average 1 in 4 (25 per cent) children will have sickle cell anaemia (β-S/β-S), 2 in 4 (50 per cent) will be carriers (β-A_1/β-S) and 1 in 4 (25 per cent) will inherit two normal β-A_1 genes. This is best illustrated diagrammatically (Fig. 5.1, where the four possible

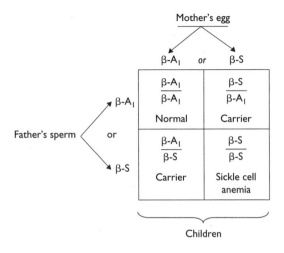

Figure 5.1 A typical recessive genetic trait

combinations of genes (their *genotype*) in the children and their phenotype are shown.

Using the same logic, it is possible to predict confidently the risk of two parents having a child with sickle cell anaemia.

- It is not possible for the children born from a normal (β-A$_1$/β-A$_1$) parent and an unaffected carrier (β-A$_1$/β-S) to have sickle cell anaemia—50 per cent will be normal (β-A$_1$/β-A$_1$) and 50 per cent will be unaffected carriers (β-A$_1$/β-S).

- It is not possible for the children born from a normal (β-A$_1$/β-A$_1$) parent and an affected parent (β-S/β-S) to have sickle cell anaemia—they will all be unaffected carriers (β-A$_1$/β-S).

- Fifty percent of the children born from a carrier parent (β-A$_1$/β-S) and an affected parent (β-S/β-S) will have sickle cell anaemia but 50 per cent will be carriers (β-A$_1$/β-S).

- One hundred per cent of the children born from two affected parents (β-S/β-S) will have sickle cell anaemia.

As individuals usually choose their partners without knowing their genetic make-up, the probability of two unaffected carriers having children with sickle cell anaemia is largely dependent on the frequency of the β-S gene mutation in the general population. As it happens, while sickle cell anaemia is lethal without treatment, β-A$_1$/β-S carriers are more resistant to malaria than normal β-A_1/β-A_1 individuals and most carriers live(d) in malaria-prone areas of the tropics. In this case, survival of the fittest has selected for a gene mutation which increases the chances of survival of 50 per cent of the (β-A_1/β-S) children, whilst sacrificing the 25 per cent that will get sickle cell anaemia. However cold-hearted, over the millennia and given the severity of malaria, the numbers of carrier children that will survive has favoured the survival of the β-S gene.

Nevertheless, studies of sickle cell anaemia in large families over several generations has consistently revealed one important characteristic of recessive inherited traits: the trait will often skip a generation as either all their carrier parents, by chance, chose normal individuals as partners or, by chance, no affected children were born of two carrier parents (the risk for each child is only 1 in 4).

Essential tremor—a dominant genetic disorder

The way ET is inherited in most of the families studied can be schematically represented by constructing a family pedigree. One such idealized pedigree is shown (Fig. 5.4) using accepted symbols for males (square) and females (circle). If the square or circle is filled, then that individual has ET; if the square or circle is empty, then that individual does not have ET. If the gene mutation is dominant, as it is in the family shown, all affected individuals have an affected parent, all children born of unaffected parents are unaffected, and affected and unaffected individuals are found in each generation. Most importantly, roughly 50 per cent of children born of an affected parent will get ET, whereas the risk of an unaffected family member passing on ET is 0 per cent.

If we call the normal gene ET^+ and the mutant gene ET^-, then a child has to inherit only one mutant ET^- gene to get ET. There is usually no history of ET in the family of the unaffected parent. It is therefore likely that the affected parent is ET^+/ET^-, and the unaffected parent is normal for both genes ET^+/ET^+. As illustrated in Fig 5.2, there is a 50 per cent chance of having a child that is affected, and the unaffected children cannot pass on ET to their children.

As in the case of sickle cell anaemia, there is the formal possibility that the observed 50 per cent of affected children could have been due to a recessive ET^- gene mutation and parental ET^-/ET^+ and ET^-/ET^- genotypes (Fig 5.3).

So how is this possibility excluded? The conclusive evidence comes from the analysis of the second generation—the children's children. For example, if each of the affected (ET^-/ET^-) children married unaffected and genetically unrelated partners with no family history of ET, there is a good chance

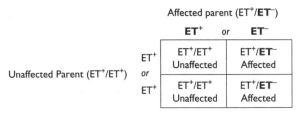

Figure 5.2 Dominant inheritance of ET

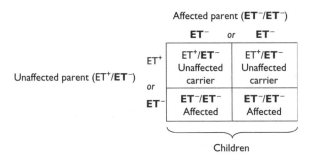

Figure 5.3 Recessive inheritance of ET

that some if not all the partners will be ET^+/ET^+. However, it is not possible for the children born from ET^+/ET^+ and **ET^-/ET^+** parents to get ET if the gene is recessive, and yet the risk of an affected parent having an affected child is always 50 per cent as shown in the pedigree (Fig 5.4). Analysis of the inheritance of ET through family pedigrees has shown that ET must be a dominant genetic trait in most of the documented families.

Personal Perspective

Being married to someone with ET, there was a 50 per cent chance that our children would inherit it. For me this was not an issue because I considered myself well informed and it was discussed openly in the family. Whilst it is a relief that our 17-year-old daughter has as yet shown no signs of ET, whilst two of her cousins have, I am now more aware of the potential implications this has on affected young people and future generations.

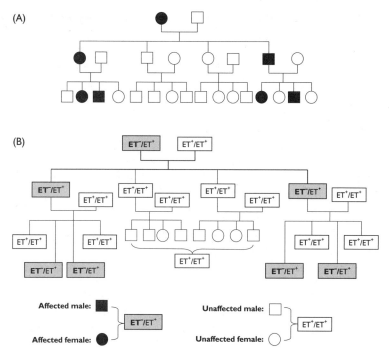

Figure 5.4 Typical ET family pedigree showing the relationship between phenotype (ET) and genotype. (A) Pedigree of a hypothetical but typical family with ET, showing males (squares) and females (circles) and whether they are affected (filled) or unaffected (open). All affected individuals have an affected parent, affected members are found in every generation, and the probability of an affected parent passing the ET on is 50 per cent. There is no risk of unaffected individuals passing on ET to their children. The gene that causes ET (ET^-) is dominant. (B) All affected individuals in the pedigree (in A) have inherited a mutant ET (ET^-) gene, whereas the unaffected members have not. It is therefore possible to assign the genotype (genetic make-up) of each individual according to whether they are affected (ET^-/ET^+) or unaffected (ET^+/ET^+).

The fact that ET is inherited as a dominant genetic trait in large families does not exclude the possibility that environment does not play a role. The way the relative contribution of genetics and environment make to a phenotype such as ET can be estimated is by analysing twins.

Twins in essential tremor—essential tremor is highly heritable

The variation in the manifestation (severity, age of onset, etc.) of ET in different individuals could be because the individuals have a different genetic background and/or because of environmental factors interacting with that genetic background. One could argue, for example, that being brought up in a family with shaking individuals in itself predisposes other family members to shake. Geneticists have therefore come up with a measure of '*heritability*' (expressed as a percentage). *Heritability* can estimate the genetic contribution to any given trait. One hundred per cent is highly heritable, 0 per cent means that it is completely environmental. One can measure it using family pedigrees (Fig. 5.4) because we know how related each family member is to every other member. The 50 per cent chance that a child born to an affected parent will be affected by ET is convincing evidence that ET is highly heritable. However, members of a family share a common environment and, whilst siblings have one half of their genes in common, they probably share 100 per cent (more or less) of their environment.

To get around the problem of the relative contribution of genes and environment to a particular disorder, twins are widely recruited in the name of genetics. Identical twins arise from a single fertilized egg (*monozygotic*) and are therefore genetically identical. In contrast, non-identical twins arose from the chance fertilization of two different eggs by two different sperm (*dizygotic*) and are therefore not genetically identical—like any other two siblings in the same family, they share only 50 per cent of their genes. Identical twins who are separated at birth are particularly informative because although they share exactly the same genes, they are brought up in different environments. Given enough identical twins separated at birth, the contribution of genes and environment to a genetic trait can be measured quite accurately. If both identical twins shake despite being brought up in different environments, genetics is a good candidate. Most twins are not separated at birth and therefore share the environment, but this applies equally to monozygotic and dizygotic twins, so any difference between the incidence of ET in monozygotic and dizygotic twins can be confidently attributed to the genes.

Identical twins are so valuable to genetic research that many countries keep a registry of twins who can be contacted by researchers and tested if they agree. The first ET twin study was carried out using the National Research Council World War II Veteran Twins Registry in the USA. A total of 196 twins aged over 65-years of age were identified with postural or kinetic tremor. Only 16 twins were available for analysis as the rest were excluded because data were only available for one twin, ET was not diagnosed, or because

Parkinson's disease was diagnosed. Of these 16, five twins were monozygotic and 11 twins were dizygotic. Both twins were diagnosed with ET in six pairs, of which three were monozygotic (3/5; 60 per cent), and three were dizygotic (3/11; 27 per cent). As about twice as many pairs of monozygotic twins (60 per cent) were affected as dizygotic (27 per cent) twins, the genes and inheritance must play a part, although the 60 per cent value in monozygotic twins is pretty low—it implies that environment contributes up to 40 per cent of the ET phenotype. There are a number of problems with this study, not least of which that it was primarily aimed at studying the genetics of Parkinson's disease, and the ET data were an incidental by-product.

A more recent Danish study was more methodical. Because ET is most evident in old age, the Danish twin registry was searched for twins aged over 70 years. A total of 2448 twins were then screened for ET using an interview and the Archimedes spiral test, and 162 twin pairs were identified that were potentially positive for ET. A total of 109 pairs were contacted and examined in more detail by a *movement disorder specialist* using tests that included drinking water with a spoon, and the finger–nose–finger test. Of the 2448 twins they started with, they ended up with 29 definite and seven probable ET. Interestingly, the incidence of ET in Denmark can be estimated using these data: 36 cases of ET out of the original total of 2448 twins they screened represents a 1.5 per cent incidence (36/2448) in the general population in Denmark. This is very close to all other general population ET incidence estimates.

Researchers were then able to ask a very simple question: how often do both identical twins shake, compared with how often do both non-identical twins shake (*concordance*)? Severity was not the issue—it was a simple yes/no answer for every pair—'Do you (both) shake?'

Of the eight Danish monozygotic twins, where at least one twin had ET, and where both twins could be examined, both twins in 8/8 cases had ET (100 per cent concordant). In contrast, of the 18 dizygotic twins, with at least one twin with ET, both twins had ET in only 3/18 (17 per cent) cases. Statistical analysis of these data yielded a heritability score for ET of 99 per cent—environment is not a factor in Denmark. For comparison, a similar study of obesity in twins revealed that only 66–70 per cent of the phenotype (obesity) is due to genetic factors—the rest is environmental (diet).

If you have ET and it runs in the family, it is 99 per cent certain that your genes are responsible. Furthermore, if you inherit the gene, it is also almost certain that you will have symptoms of ET by the age of 65–70, so the trait is highly '*penetrant*'. However complex your relationship with members of your family is/was/will be, the relationship(s) do not have a significant impact on whether you shake or not—it is in your genes.

Identifying the essential tremor genes

Familial cases of ET can be exploited to try and identify the genes that cause it. Consider the same hypothetical pedigree used before (Fig. 5.4) where we are certain that ET was transmitted through the grandmother's side of the family, and the presence of affected individuals in three generations is taken as strong evidence that it is a dominant trait. As the affected parents have affected and unaffected offspring (1:1 ratio), the affected parents must have one normal ET^+ gene and one mutant ET^- gene, whereas the unaffected parents must have two normal ET^+ genes. We can thus allocate the genotype to each family member. There are a number of affected (ET^-/ET^+) and unaffected (ET^+/ET^+) members of the family, and each affected individual inherited the ET^- gene from their affected (ET^-/ET^+) parent who in turn inherited the same ET^- gene from the (ET^-/ET^+) grandmother. Conversely, unaffected (ET^+/ET^+) family members cannot have inherited the ET^- gene from the grandmother.

For the sake of argument, let us assume that the ET gene is on chromosome 2. Grandmother had one ET^- **chromosome 2** and one ET^+ chromosome 2, and had a 50 per cent chance of passing on one or the other chromosome 2 to each of her children. Affected members of the family will have inherited the ET^- **chromosome 2** derived (directly or indirectly) from grandmother, and the unaffected family members may have inherited the ET^+ chromosome 2 (directly or indirectly) but cannot have inherited the ET^- **chromosome 2** from the grandmother. This can then be added to the pedigree (Fig. 5.4B)

DNA fingerprinting can be used to tell which chromosome, and more specifically which part of a chromosome, a particular DNA sequence came from. Fingerprinting can distinguish between both of the father's chromosome 2s, and can distinguish both of the mother's chromosome 2s from each other, and distinguish between mother's and father's chromosome 2s. The hypothetical pedigree can therefore become very informative as the origin of every single chromosome 2 in every individual in a large family pedigree can be traced by fingerprinting.

All the affected individuals will have their grandmother's ET^- **chromosome 2**, whereas none of the unaffected relatives (open symbols) have, and it can be traced back through two generations of affected family members to the grandmother. If a similar analysis was carried out with all 23 chromosomes, and only the grandmother's **chromosome 2** consistently appeared in affected but not unaffected relatives, one could be reasonably certain that grandmother's ET^- gene in this family was somewhere on chromosome 2. As there are 30 000 genes spread out across the 23 chromosomes, the mapping of the **ET** gene to chromosome 2 narrows down the search to identify the actual gene to roughly 30 000/23 = 1300 genes.

We inherit half of our chromosomes from our father and half from our mother, who in turn inherited half their chromosomes from each of their parents. This implies that a quarter of our chromosomes are identical to those in each of our four grandparents. If this was the case, and chromosomes were passed on to offspring more or less unchanged, the genetic and phenotypic diversity we observe in human beings (we are all so different) would be significantly less than is observed—we would all be much more closely related genetically to each other. However, the chromosomes and genes are 'mixed' during the production of the haploid eggs or sperm in a process called *meiosis*. It is during meiosis that chromosome mixing occurs in a process called *meiotic recombination*. The word *recombination* literally means that information between chromosome pairs is exchanged to give hybrid chromosomes.

There are four possible products for each of the 23 chromosomes during meiosis, and each product assorts at random into any one egg or sperm. Despite the mixing of genes at the level of the chromosomes, the overall chance of passing on one or the other of the parental genes to a child remains at 50 per cent.

The added complexity of recombination during meiosis is incredibly useful in medical genetics. We can simplify the ET pedigree as we are only interested in relatives who inherited some or all of grandmother's **chromosome 2**. Because we know where specific pieces of DNA sequences map on any particular chromosome, we can precisely map which bit of **chromosome 2** any affected or unaffected individual inherited.

By aligning the recombinant and non-recombinant chromosome 2s that contain some or all of grandmother's original **chromosome 2**, and comparing affected and unaffected relatives within this pedigree, one can ask the simple question: which bit of grandmother's **chromosome 2** is present in all affected individuals, but is absent in all unaffected individuals? As illustrated in Fig. 5.5, the same region (carrying the *) between the two dotted lines is inherited by all affected individuals but not by unaffected individuals. The ET gene (*) maps somewhere in between the two dotted lines and represents 10 per cent of the whole of chromosome 2 (for example). Mapping the ET gene to chromosome 2 first reduced the number of possible ET genes from 30 000 to roughly 1300 genes. The further fine mapping of the ET gene to an interval on chromosome 2 between the dotted line has reduced the number of possible genes to about 130. This genetic approach to fine mapping a gene can be applied to one particularly large family, or to several (unrelated) families to increase the statistical power and resolution of the analysis.

This approach has been employed to try and identify the gene(s) involved in ET families, and a pattern is beginning to emerge as results are independently

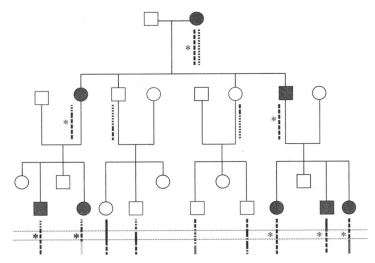

Figure 5.5 Mapping ET genes. This pedigree shows only the bits of the grandmother's original chromosome 2 that carries the dominant ET-causing gene mutation (*). The parental origin of each part of each chromosome 2 and each part of that chromosome can be determined by fingerprinting, and can be mapped in affected and unaffected individuals. Alignment of the chromosomes, and a comparison of affected and unaffected individuals, shows that all affected individuals contain that part of grandmother's chromosome 2 that has the *, whereas unaffected individuals do not. The ET susceptibility locus has thus been mapped to that chromosomal interval that lies between the dotted lines.

reproduced. If a mutation in a single gene is always responsible for ET, genetic association studies should always give the same result (one gene or chromosomal interval) irrespective of the ethnic or geographic origins of the ET families. If more than one gene can cause ET, the actual mutated gene in any one ET family will depend to a certain extent on their genetic background. Populations which are most ethnically and geographically similar/related may share the same gene mutation, whereas another distinct population (assuming little historical interbreeding) might share a mutation in a different gene, and this is what has been found.

One study of Icelandic families mapped an ET gene (*ETM1*; *ET Mutated gene 1*) to a region of DNA on chromosome 3. This was confirmed by a Russian study which also found that *ETM1* was linked to ET in four Tajic families. In contrast, the analysis of a large Czech American family, mapped a second independent ET susceptibility *locus* (*ETM2*) to chromosome 2, and this has been confirmed by the analysis of three unrelated American families (non-Czech) and Singaporean ET families of Chinese descent. The evidence that more than one gene mutation can cause ET is therefore very strong. Furthermore, the Russian study identified one family where ET was definitely not linked to either *ETM1* or *ETM2*, and similar negative results were obtained in the analysis of a large six generation family in Midwestern USA and in studies of Italian familial cases of ET. The only explanation is that other genes, in addition to *ETM1* and *ETM2*, have yet to be identified.

Although a number of genes within the *ETM1* and *ETM2* chromosomal intervals are very plausible candidates (the proteins encoded are involved in nerve cell function), the identity of the actual gene(s) that cause ET has yet to be confirmed, but this should happen in the near future.

Essential tremor is a complex inherited disorder

The genetic association studies of ET families have shown that mutations in a number of genes can cause ET. However, whilst the highly heritable and dominant mode of inheritance of ET in most large families studied is obvious, simple genetics does not explain the sporadic ET cases, nor does it explain why the age of onset and tremor severity can vary so widely.

In sporadic cases of ET, the absence of a family history has been attributed to the environment because the documented studies suggest that ET is a dominant genetic trait. However, an alternative possibility is that ET can, in some instances, be inherited as a recessive genetic trait, as this is more difficult to detect in family trees. There is evidence from other inherited disorders such as Parkinson's disease that different mutations in different genes can cause the same disorder, and that some of these mutations are dominant and some recessive. The chances of two unaffected (ET^-/ET^+) carriers having affected children (ET^-/ET^-) are only 1 in 4, so in small families this recessive trait can be difficult to detect—the chances of two affected children in the same family is 1 in 16. Similarly, the probability of two carriers meeting and having children is dependent on the frequency of that gene in the general population, so rarer gene mutations will again be more difficult to detect in family trees. Nevertheless, the possibility of a recessive inheritance in some cases of ET cannot be excluded and, together with the known multiple dominant gene mutations, underlines the genetic complexity of the disorder.

We have also already seen how males and females are equally likely to get ET; it is not *sex-linked,* as this would implicate the X or Y chromosome. However, we have also already mentioned the fact that there are data suggesting that males (XY chromosomes) are twice as likely to show early symptoms of ET in childhood than females (XX chromosomes), whereas females are six times more likely to develop head tremor than men. These gender-dependent differences in the manifestation of ET can be attributed to the sex-determining X or Y chromosomes—females have twice as many X chromosomes as males. The Y chromosome is relatively small and contains a small numbers of genes, most of which are involved in sex determination, so sex-linked genetic disorders are usually due to gene mutations on the X chromosome. It is therefore likely that there are genes on the X chromosome which can modify the progression/manifestation of the ET caused by the inheritance of the ET-causing gene on one of the other (non-sex) chromosomes. For example, males that inherit an ET-causing mutation on chromosome 2 or 3 which will cause ET in middle age, but also inherit a mutated gene on the X chromosome from their mother, are predisposed to early onset ET in childhood—in contrast, early-onset ET in females may require that they inherit two mutated copies of the genes on the X chromosome (it is recessive). ET females that inherit two copies of a mutated gene on the X chromosome are predisposed to head tremor.

Other genes on other chromosomes (dominant or recessive) could equally contribute to the manifestation of the ET symptoms so, in addition to the ET-causing genes, there are a number of other genes that affect the progression and manifestation of ET.

Genetic testing in essential tremor

Let us imagine the future. Mutations in at least 10 different genes are responsible for ET, and these were identified as a result of countless genetic association studies and the sequencing of countless candidate genes. The physics, chemistry, electrochemistry, biology and biochemistry of the proteins encoded by the normal and mutant genes have been elucidated, and we have a very good idea of how and why the tremor in ET is essential. We are left with one last question. So what? The answer will have to address at least two distinct issues: firstly, what is the scientific value of the discovery? Secondly, how does this help the average person affected by ET?

There is no doubt that the identification of the ET genes will help elucidate the workings of the brain so, from a scientific point of view, the expense and effort can be easily justified. The identification of the genes, how they are mutated, and what the encoded protein does in the living brain, represent major advances in our understanding of the exact biochemical defects that lead to a disease. Furthermore, we can begin to address fundamental questions about the potential relationship between, for example, Parkinson's disease and ET. If the same genes are defective in the two disorders, then the disorders themselves are genetically related and share a common genetically determined risk factor. This has been studied and, to date, Parkinson's disease and ET are genetically *unrelated*.

In the long term, this understanding may well lead to the development of designer drugs that specifically target the particular biochemical defect. Laboratories and pharmaceutical companies all over the world are trying to develop drugs that will specifically halt the progressive brain damage found in Alzheimer's and Parkinson's disease patients, but it would not cure or reverse the disease. However, with a few highly successful exceptions such as haemophilia and diabetes, the promise of designer drugs based on the knowledge of the biochemical defect in more complex inherited diseases has yet to bear fruit. On the whole, the therapies still target the symptoms rather than the cause of the disease—cystic fibrosis (CF) remains fatal despite the discovery of the CF gene in 1989.

From the patient's point of view, the value of knowing which particular gene is mutated depends on the disease, its severity, and whether a treatment is available that can either prevent or slow down the progression of the disease. Most would agree that the early diagnosis of congenital disorders that can be treated and will allow treatment to begin before irreversible damage has been caused is desirable, and would increase the effectiveness of that treatment. Prevention is better than a cure—it is far better to diagnose a haemophiliac before they start bleeding, and diagnose diabetics before they fall into a coma. Genetic testing can be carried out as soon after birth as necessary (a drop of blood is all that is needed), and therapy commenced whenever it is clinically required, or, individuals can also be monitored throughout life. Treatment can involve taking medication, or may simply require a change of lifestyle and/or diet to improve life expectancy and quality of life significantly. A genetic test might influence the choice of therapy, but that is usually not necessary in ET as alternative diagnostic tools are available (Chapter 3).

Regrettably there are a large number of inherited diseases where there is no cure or effective treatment available—and this includes ET. The symptoms can be treated, but progression cannot be slowed or stopped. In these cases, the role of genetic testing is quite different—at a very crude level, the testing can be used to prevent children who would carry these disorders from being conceived or born. For example, CF is a recessive trait, and roughly 1 in 22 White Americans are carriers of the mutant CF gene (CF^+/CF^-); if two carriers have a child, there will be a 25 per cent chance that the child will get CF and die in early adulthood—a particularly distressing life and a highly unpleasant death. Because the CF gene is known, potential parents with a history of CF in their family(ies) can be tested for CF gene mutations. If neither parent is a carrier, or if only one is a carrier, there is absolutely no risk of them having a CF child and they can safely breed. However, if both turn out to be carriers they then face a very difficult decision as their options are limited. Many will believe that a 25 per cent risk is a risk worth taking and will let nature take its course. Others believe that they have no right to interfere with nature. However, having to watch your CF child suffer and die is an horrendous prospect, and one that many carriers will wish to avoid for the child's sake as well as their own. The only realistic option open to these couples is prenatal genetic testing.

In amniocentesis, which is usually carried out at the 16th week of pregnancy, a syringe is inserted through the abdominal wall and through the uterine wall to collect cells from the amniotic fluid surrounding the fetus. The fetal cells can then be analysed for gene mutations. If the fetus turns out to carry two mutant CF genes (CF^-/CF^-), the only option left is to terminate the pregnancy—at 16 weeks this is a harrowing and highly undesirable experience in itself. Chorionic villus sampling of a fetus can take place earlier in a pregnancy (8–10 weeks), but in both cases the sampling procedure itself carries a small risk to mother and fetus. The only remaining option is *in vitro* fertilization (IVF) where sperm is used to fertilize eggs in a test tube. As the fertilized eggs divide and reach the 6- to 10-cell stage, a single cell is removed and tested. Only CF^+/CF^+ embryos are transferred back into the uterus and allowed to develop to full term.

Ultimately, a genetic test is only worth considering if the genetic information can be used in a meaningful way to prevent suffering and/or increase the quality of life. In the absence of either a cure or effective therapies that will slow the progression of so many inherited disorders, genetic testing currently has one main purpose—to help potential at-risk parents decide on whether to have children or not, and/or whether to terminate pregnancies. The pros and cons of genetic tests have to be weighed very carefully, and will vary between individuals and between diseases—it is a moral and ethical question.

At present, a genetic test for ET would be of little practical use. As a conclusive diagnosis of ET can be difficult, a genetic test might help confirm a diagnosis if the test was positive and thus exclude other neurological disorders. This in turn would reduce the need for further investigation and could also potentially influence therapeutic choices. As therapeutic options are limited, this would be of little clinical import. If a genetic test was negative, however, it would be inconclusive, as other as yet unidentified ET genes may or may not exist. Ultimately, assuming that somewhere in the region of 10 ET genes exist, each and every gene would need to be screened for a mutation in every affected family member. Furthermore, the genes that could cause conditions that were similar to ET might also have to be screened for mutations. The financial implications of such a screening programme need to be taken into account—at this moment in time, a cost–benefit analysis would probably conclude that valuable resources would be better spent on refining and improving existing treatments and/or spent on research into new treatments, but this might change over time.

We would not wish to influence anybody's decision if a genetic test for ET were one day to become available—genetic counselling is usually offered. However, the key question is whether life with ET is unbearable. How many people with ET are unable to lead a reasonably normal and productive life? Are prospective parents prepared to undergo amniocentesis with its associated dangers, and consider abortion to avoid having a child with ET? Is the knowledge that we carry a mutation in a particular ET gene of any practical use? Even if we do carry the gene mutation, this may not tell us the age of onset or severity of ET in any child that did inherit it. After all that, in a worse case scenario of severe ET, the symptoms can be treated. ET couples considering having children today also have the advantage of knowing that given the rapid progress in medicine, a better treatment, or even cure, for ET may have been discovered well before the prospective child's ET becomes a serious disability.

ET can be difficult, but it is not unbearable, and effective therapies are available.

6 Possible causes of essential tremor

As already discussed, there are a number of reasons to believe that there will not be a single cause of ET—no single mutant gene or aberrant neuron will be shared by all affected individuals. Other than the characteristic postural and kinetic tremor, everything else in ET is highly variable. The high incidence of ET worldwide makes it extremely unlikely that all affected individuals have the same genetic defect, and this is supported by the preliminary mapping of at least two different ET susceptibility genes, with many more yet to come (Chapter 5).

Although ET can be thought of as a family of distinct movement disorders, an alternative is to think of voluntary movement being under the control of a complex nerve cell network, or circuit, involving many regions of the brain. A defect anywhere in that network will potentially affect the fine control of voluntary movement and give rise to ET. Whilst each defect or deficiency affects the same tremorogenic neuronal circuit, the other highly variable ET-associated symptoms will depend in part on where in the network the particular ET-causing defect occurred, and the nature of the defect itself.

A basic understanding of which parts of the brain are implicated in ET and how voluntary movement is controlled is needed before considering what that tremor-causing pathway might be, together with a brief description of the way muscles are controlled during voluntary movement.

Essential tremor as a neurological disorder of the central nervous system

The bilateral postural and kinetic tremor that is so characteristic of ET could, in principle, be a disorder in any of the physiological processes that control muscle contraction. In other words, there could be something wrong with the muscles themselves, or something wrong with the nerves between the muscle and the spinal cord, or the spinal cord itself, or any one of the different areas of the brain involved in the control of voluntary movement. All the evidence suggests that the defect that causes ET is in the central nervous system. Perhaps the clearest evidence is the fact that whilst alcohol consumption will reduce tremor severity in ET, injection of alcohol directly into the arm has no influence on the tremor in the arm—the anti-tremor effects of alcohol must therefore be acting indirectly in the central nervous system.

Several areas of the brain are involved in the control of movement, and movement disorders such as ET and Parkinson's disease are clearly the result of a defect in one or more of these key parts of the brain. Studies of Parkinson's disease in particular, but also indirect evidence from ET, have implicated the cortex, the cerebellum, the brainstem, the thalamus, and/or the basal ganglia in the tremors. The central nervous system can be represented as a hierarchical structure leading from the 'thinking' part of the brain, the cortex, through to the motor and sensory neurons in the brainstem and spinal cord. Nevertheless, all of these regions of the brain have to communicate with each other to control voluntary movement, so in many ways it is perhaps best to consider them as a regulatory circuit.

Cortex: plans, initiates and controls voluntary movement.

Basal ganglia: involved in fine-tuning and learning movement.

Thalamus: monitors movement as reported by the senses. Compares movement with the original instructions sent by the cortex and reports back to the cortex.

Cerebellum: fine-tuning and monitoring movement as reported by the senses.

Brainstem: conduit for information between the brain, the senses, and the muscles.

Spinal cord: conduit for information between the brain, the senses, and the muscles below the head.

If the origin of the 4–12 Hz electrical activity detected in the muscles of the shaking arm by EMG is the central nervous system, then a rhythmic neuronal activity, or other evidence, should also be detected in the brain during postural or kinetic tremor. There are two main lines of evidence.

Tremor-related nerve cell activity

We have already seen that tremor-related nerve cell activity (TRA) in the Vim is found in the thalamus (Chapter 4) and there is a linear relationship between nerve cell firing in the Vim in the thalamus and the ET tremor-related EMG recordings (4–12 Hz) in the muscles of the arm. About one-third of the nerve cells in the Vim fire at this TRA frequency, thus enabling the tracing of oscillating nerve impulses in the arm to individual nerve cells in a specific region of the brain.

The discovery of nerve cells that have TRA in the same region (Vim) of the thalamus that is destroyed (thalamotomy) or stimulated (deep brain stimulation) to treat ET (Chapter 4) is very gratifying and it would be very convenient to believe that the aberrant thalamic activity is solely responsible for the 4–12 Hz EMG electrical activity in the shaking arms of people with ET. Unfortunately, this does not prove that the thalamic TRA nerve cells are the actual source or origin of the tremor. The complex neural circuitry and regulatory loops connecting the thalamus to the cortex, the cerebellum, the basal ganglia and the brainstem means that the TRA detected in the thalamus may be a symptom of a defect elsewhere in the central nervous system. There is thus the formal possibility that an independent oscillating nerve cell activity could be responsible for both the EMG-related activity in the shaking arms and the periodic firing of thalamic cells.

Imaging studies of the brain in essential tremor

The activity in the human ET brain at rest and during postural tremor has been analysed using functional imaging techniques to try and fine-map specific regions of the brain that are affected during tremor. Increased nerve cell activity requires energy expenditure, and this in turn requires a local increase in the blood supply. Imaging techniques such as positron emission tomography (PET) and functional magnetic resonance imaging (fMRI) are able to monitor changes in blood flow to specific regions of the brain which is taken as a sign of increased requirement for blood-borne oxygen and nutrients that are associated with increased nerve cell activity. A number of such studies have consistently found increased nerve cell activity in the cerebellum, the cortex and the thalamus, but did not find a tremor-related increase in blood supply to the brainstem.

Muscle contraction

Movement of a finger or arm is a complex process involving the communication of instructions from the brain to the appropriate muscles. However, a muscle can only contract or relax—one muscle can move a finger in one direction (*agonist*), but a different muscle is needed to bring the finger back to its original position (*antagonist*). The importance of opposing muscles is nicely illustrated by considering the crocodile who has powerful muscles to shut (bite) its jaw, but has no opposing muscles to open the jaw—it relies on gravity to open its mouth and the lower jaw literally drops.

Prolonged contraction of agonist and antagonist muscles at the same time (co-contraction) leads to a sustained abnormal posture, slower movements and pain (*dystonia*).

The signals from the brain that initiate voluntary movement are communicated to the muscles by electrical signals that travel through nerve cells, but a nerve cell can transmit either an *excitatory* signal or an *inhibitory* signal; it cannot transmit both (Chapter 4), and the signal can only travel in one direction. The brain is not connected directly to the muscles—it is connected directly to the spinal column by '*efferent*' neurons in the 'pyramidal pathway', and motor neurons connect the spinal cord to the muscles. The nervous system is thus subdivided into the *central nervous system*, which comprises the brain and spinal cord, and the *peripheral nervous system*, linking the central nervous system to the rest of the body.

An excitatory signal that triggers agonist muscle contraction must also tell the opposing antagonist muscle to relax but, as muscles will relax in the absence of an excitatory signal, antagonist muscle relaxation is achieved by preventing an excitatory signal reaching the muscle if it is already relaxed, or switching off an excitatory signal. For a single brain signal to control both agonist and antagonist muscles, the excitatory ($+$) signal from the brain to the agonist muscles thus has to be converted to an inhibitory negative ($-$) signal to the antagonist muscles to prevent co-contraction. The negative signal to the antagonist muscles is not so much a signal in its own right, but rather a signal to prevent (inhibit) an excitatory signal reaching the relaxed antagonist muscle.

As illustrated in Fig. 6.1, both the agonist and antagonist muscles are connected to separate excitatory nerves from the brain as they both have to be able to respond to excitatory signals. However, an excitatory nerve to the agonist muscle is also connected to an inhibitory nerve, which in turn is connected to the excitatory nerve to the antagonist muscle. When the brain fires an excitatory ($+$) signal to the agonist, the nerve also activates an inhibitory ($-$) signal that stops or blocks any excitatory signals reaching the antagonist muscles, keeping them relaxed.

The principles of voluntary movement

Controlled movement also requires fine-tuning to tell muscles how far to contract to achieve the requested movement (force, speed and direction), and this involves continuous monitoring by the senses and corrections as necessary. As a typist writes a sentence on the computer keyboard, the brain thinks of the words to be typed and sends signals to one of the fingers.

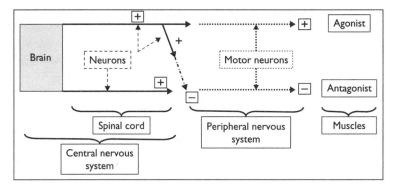

Figure 6.1 Nerves and muscle contraction. Simplified representation of the central nervous system that comprises the brain and spinal cord, and the peripheral nervous system that uses motor neurons to connect to the agonist and antagonist muscles. If an excitatory (——▶+) signal is sent by the brain to an agonist muscle to contract, that signal is converted into an inhibitory signal (−) using an inhibitory nerve cell (interneuron·····▶) signal to the motor neuron connecting to the antagonist muscle. This prevents an excitatory signal reaching the antagonist muscle which stays relaxed, and thus prevents co-contraction.

Agonist muscles in the appropriate finger in the appropriate hand will contract to press the right key, and antagonist muscles reverse the movement to lift the finger off the keyboard. Typing is also controlled by eyesight, and even the sense of touch has a role to make sure that the right finger presses the right key and that the correct letter has been registered by the computer and appears on the screen. The senses are therefore critical in setting the target for the planning and execution of a particular movement.

Blind people can lead relatively normal lives, and sighted people are not completely disabled in darkness, so eyesight is not a pre-requisite for manual dexterity or any other motor skills. We are all aware of the position of our body parts relative both to each other and to the immediate environment, and can use that information to initiate and control complex movement. In addition to the senses, there is a two-way communication between the muscles and the brain. The precise (relative) position of a muscle is communicated to the brain which is thus informed about where the muscle is, what it is doing and, in the case of the voluntary movement it has initiated, how that movement is progressing. Like the more obvious senses of touch, sight, hearing and smell, we can 'sense' the position of our body parts.

Voluntary movement implies that the brain is involved in initiating and controlling that movement. However, the degree to which the 'brain' is involved does vary according to which muscles are involved. When we decide to walk across the room, it is a conscious decision, but we do not consciously control each step of each leg once that decision has been made, and do not have to think about which leg is moving at each step. Once we have learnt to walk in early childhood, and that is mainly a question of balance, the only conscious input we have to make during locomotion is to avoid obstacles which we can see or feel. Even when we do trip, regaining our balance or breaking the fall is a matter of our reflexes. Walking is therefore largely automatic although input from the brain fine-tunes the movement.

Another motor skill that is voluntarily controlled but is learnt in early childhood is speech. We are not conscious of the vocal cord muscles used in talking, but the basic skills have to be learnt. In addition to the instructions from the brain to say particular words, speech is also controlled by feedback information from the vocal cord muscles themselves (including vibrations as sound is produced) and from our hearing so that the volume, pitch, etc. of the sounds generated can be modulated as circumstances dictate. However, like locomotion, once the basic skills have been learnt, the actual muscular movements involved are largely automatic, and minimal conscious input from the brain is required.

The voluntary muscles we use most in the body are those that move the eyeballs. We are continually looking around and scanning our environment, and this involves instructions from the brain telling our eyes (and head) to move so that they focus on a particular object. Pretty much all eye movement is voluntary, and therefore controlled by the brain, but we are not conscious of the precise muscular movements required to point the eyes in a certain direction, and are completely unaware of how the movement of the two eyes is co-ordinated so that they both focus on the same object. Unlike speech and locomotion, the use of our eyes is not learnt—it is instinctive despite the fact that it is under voluntary control.

In contrast, the use of the arms, wrists and fingers is almost completely consciously controlled by the brain and is continually being modulated by information fed back to the brain by the senses. Unlike the legs and eyes, there is no automatic co-ordination of movement of the two arms as they can independently perform quite different operations. The movements we ask our upper limbs to perform are never quite the same—they are unique and, therefore, on the whole, are not learnt in the same way that we learn to use other voluntary muscles. There are exceptions—manual dexterity does improve with practice, and this applies in particular to repetitive actions such as typing, working on an assembly line, or playing a musical instrument.

However, these repetitive movements represent a relatively small proportion of the actions we demand of our arms/wrists/fingers. The bulk of this voluntary movement is under the direct control of the brain; we can see and feel the muscles moving, and are therefore very conscious of that movement.

Thus there is a large activity-dependent variation in the input required from the brain to control voluntary movement. Much of what appears to be voluntary is to a certain extent automatic and/or learnt. It is also worth remembering that the postural and kinetic tremor in ET does not affect all voluntary muscles equally. Tremor of the arms/hands is shared by all ET patients, whereas shaking of the head and/or voice is less common and is related to the severity of the tremor in the arms. Shaking legs is rare in 'classical' ET, and this immediately suggests that the susceptibility of any one muscle to ET-related tremor is directly or indirectly related to the input required from the brain to initiate and control the movement of that muscle. The tremor in ET during voluntary movement thus implies that the defect involves the communication between those 'higher' (cognitive) regions of the brain involved in planning and executing movement, and the muscles.

The thalamus and the control of voluntary movement

The brain can be subdivided into anatomically and functionally defined regions. For example, our ability to think relies on the processing of information in the cerebral cortex on the outside of the brain, and there are specific regions within the cortex that process information from the senses (e.g. visual cortex for sight), or that are involved in initiating and controlling voluntary movement (motor cortex). However, the control of voluntary movement by the cortex is not a simple question of sending a signal to the muscles (via the peripheral nervous system), as it is a complex process that includes fine-tuning and feedback from the senses that are monitoring the execution of the movement, and this requires a regulatory network.

The information from all the senses except smell, and this includes sensory information from nerves below the head (somatosensory), passes through the thalamus on the way to the cortex. For example, somatosensory signals travel up the spinal cord and brainstem, and connect directly, or indirectly via the cerebellum, to the thalamus (*ventral posterior lateral* nucleus) and then on to the cortex. Similarly, light, movement and colour are detected by specific nerve cells in the retina (rods and cones) of the eye and these stimuli are converted into electrical signals that are transmitted to the brain. The electrical signals from the eyes first arrive in the thalamus (*lateral geniculate nucleus*) before being projected to the visual cortex. The thalamus therefore plays a central role in the control of voluntary movement.

There is also evidence that many of the cortex nerve cells that connect to motor structures such as the brainstem and spinal cord have branches that connect to the thalamus.

When the 'higher order' regions of the brain cortex involved in cognitive functions decide to initiate movement, the decision is sent down the brain to the spinal cord and then on to motor neurons in the peripheral nervous system. However, the thalamus receives a 'copy' of the instructions sent out by the motor cortex, and then sends the instructions back to higher cortical areas to keep the cortex informed about the precise instructions that had been sent to motor centres to plan or execute movement. It also relays information from the senses to the cortex to help monitor the progress of the planned movement. The thalamus is thus a critical interface between information travelling from the cortex to the motor centres, and from the senses back to the cortex, and is therefore involved in many aspects of the initiation and control of movement. The control of muscle movement (motor output) thus requires a series of regulatory feedback loops with the thalamus as a central monitoring station (Figure 6.2).

The sheer volume and diversity of information that passes through the thalamus during voluntary movement is astonishing, particularly as that information is processed before being relayed on to other parts of the brain. As a primary recipient of all information from the senses except smell, it plays a key role in keeping the cortex informed about the rest of the body and its relationship to the environment. Similarly, it receives a copy of most of the instructions sent out to the muscles by the motor cortex, and compares the movement planned by the cortex with the execution of that movement as reported by the senses. Most importantly, there is a direct relationship between thalamic neuronal activity to the motor cortex and the control of movement. If communication between the thalamus and the cortex is stimulated (excitatory), movement is facilitated, whereas suppression (inhibitory) of thalamic activity suppresses movement.

Linking tremor and anxiety in essential tremor

It is not immediately obvious how a nerve cell defect that causes tremor during voluntary movement can also specifically affect anxiety. As alluded to in Chapters 2 and 4, the thalamus also has direct connections with the part of the brain that is critically involved in controlling emotion, and anxiety and fear in particular—the *amygdala*.

Most sensory information, including the sensory information about potential or actual danger, travels to the thalamus before being relayed to the cortex. However, the thalamus also connects directly to the amygdala so that sensory information that requires a rapid response (fear in particular) can be acted upon immediately. This is the '*fight or flight*' response to danger.

A loud frightening noise is detected by the auditory cells in the ear which signal the thalamus. The thalamus relays that signal to the cortex so that the auditory information can be integrated with all the other sensory (e.g. sight) and cognitive information received by the brain and come up with an appropriate response. In an emergency, this whole process is relatively slow, so a more rapid immediate response is required. The thalamus also sends a copy of the auditory information received from the ears to the amygdala (Figure 6.2). Processing of this information in the thalamus and amygdala swiftly decides whether the sensory input constitutes a threat. If a threat is perceived, the amygdala signals to other regions of the brain which activate the emotional response systems—this will cause rapid breathing, a racing heart, sweating, etc., but also triggers hormonal responses including adrenaline release by the adrenal gland (the adrenaline rush). Significantly, one of the most effective drugs in the treatment of ET is the 'beta-blocker' propranolol (Chapter 4) which dampens or blocks the downstream consequences of the (β-adrenergic) activation of the 'flight or fight' response.

If there is a defect in the ET thalamus, it might have an indirect knock-on effect on the function of the amygdala. The thalamic signals sent to the amygdala may be stronger than normal and thus unnecessarily trigger the 'fight or flight' response in the amygdala. ET patients might be hypersensitive to sensory input and will therefore be prone to anxiety—they will understandably seek to avoid situations that trigger the emotional response. This stress response must be tightly regulated or we would all be in a continual state of fear—there must be some threshold below which signals received by the amygdala from the senses do not trigger this stress response. The concept of a threshold is supported by the observation that the threshold is not fixed and can vary considerably. When we are already frightened, that threshold is lowered and we become hypersensitive to sensory input (disconcerted by an unexpected but not particularly loud sound, for example). Furthermore, emotional responses can be learnt. We can enjoy a firework display even though, if not expected or out of context, the same noise would trigger the 'fight or flight' rapid reaction. Similarly, if a non-threatening sound is often accompanied shortly thereafter by something unpleasant (an electrical shock), we learn to associate the non-threatening sound with the unpleasant and the sound will itself eventually trigger the 'fight or flight' response when we hear it.

The neural network and the control of voluntary movement

Thalamic communication with the motor cortex is subject to control by other regions of the brain such as the basal ganglia and cerebellum, which either stimulate (cerebellum) or suppress (basal ganglia) thalamic activity and thus facilitate or suppress movement.

The activities of the basal ganglia and cerebellum are themselves regulated by other regions of the brain and brainstem, so thalamic neuronal communication with the motor cortex is ultimately determined by the overall balance of the excitatory and inhibitory signals it receives from a variety of sources, including the cortex itself. Thus, despite its central role in the regulation of the motor cortex, the thalamus is but one part of a larger

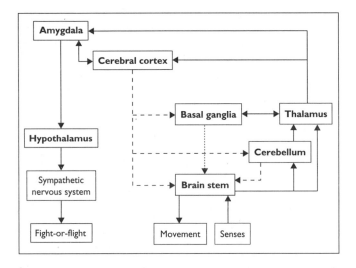

Figure 6.2 The neural circuit in voluntary movement. Simplified representation of the complex interconnections between different parts of the brain that are involved in initiating and monitoring (the senses) the execution of voluntary movement planned by the cerebral cortex. The main input into the cerebral cortex comes from the thalamus which is in turn controlled by the brainstem, cerebellum, and basal ganglia. In principle, a defect anywhere in this network could cause either tremor or difficulty in movement. The link between the thalamus and the amygdala which controls emotion, and in particular the 'fight or flight response via the hypothalamus and the sympathetic nervous system, is shown.

regulatory neuronal network, and it is the overall activity of that network that ultimately determines whether movement is facilitated or suppressed by the motor cortex. Similarly, because all of these regions of the brain are interconnected, and there is no obvious or consistent sign of specific neurodegeneration or damage in the ET brain, the origin/cause of the thalamic tremor-related activity (TRA) could in principle be anywhere in that neuronal network (Fig. 6.2). The concept of a network as a functional entity in movement control probably best represents the interdependent cerebral regulatory pathways that ultimately control movement, and is thus consistent with the data implicating more than one region of the brain in ET.

The amygdala has been included in the network as it has been implicated in emotion and the 'fight or flight' response to danger, and the thalamus does relay somatosensory information to the amygdala and therefore is involved in controlling amygdala function. The amygdala is therefore susceptible to any defect in the neural network that regulates the activity of the thalamus, whether the defect is in the thalamus itself or in the other regions of the neural network that controls voluntary movement.

Essential tremor may be a deficit of inhibitory (GABA) neurotransmitter

As ET is a hyperkinetic movement disorder, it is tempting to speculate that the tremor is a result of an excess of excitatory thalamic activity which is communicated to the motor cortex and then on to the muscles during voluntary movement. Clinical interventions to relieve the symptoms of ET rely on drugs that act generally within the central nervous system, or indirectly to block the 'fight or flight' response by the autonomic nervous system. Because the medical therapies do not specifically target any one region of the brain, they have general and non-specific effects within the central nervous system

Some of the drugs that act in the brain and are used to treat ET increase inhibitory (GABA agonists) nerve cell activity (Chapter 4). For the sake of argument, let us assume that the excess activity in ET is due to a deficiency in inhibitory nerve cell activity—the balance between excitatory and inhibitory signals in the thalamus is disrupted in favour of excitatory (hyperkinetic) activity. This excess of thalamic activity could equally be due to a deficiency of inhibitory nerve cell activity in the basal ganglia or cerebellum, as they control thalamic activity. As the basal ganglia, cerebellum and thalamus are all part of, and contribute to, the overall balance of excitatory and inhibitory activity in the network that controls voluntary movement, an inhibitory nerve cell deficiency in any one (or more) component of the network will have very similar overall effects on the control of movement.

However, GABA is a very important inhibitory neurotransmitter that is used widely throughout the central nervous system, and any general deficiency in GABA activity would have widespread effects on brain function. Yet the main symptoms of ET are largely limited to a postural/kinetic tremor. Many of these drugs bind to—and activate—GABA receptors on postsynaptic neurons, thus enhancing the inhibitory effects normally induced by GABA. However, many of these chemicals are highly neurotoxic and are used socially or in the clinic at sublethal doses that maximize the 'benefits' and minimize the damage/side-effects. The absence of GABA would be lethal, and a slight general deficiency in GABA activity would have greater consequences on the function of the central nervous system than is actually observed in ET. Conversely, a defect that affected GABA clearance from the synaptic cleft would be a GABA agonist and might have effects that resemble chronic alcohol intoxication

To understand how the effects of a GABA deficiency might be limited within the central nervous system, we need to consider not the GABA neurotransmitter, but the GABA receptor on the postsynaptic cell.

The GABA receptor

There are two main types of GABA receptors, $GABA_A$ and $GABA_B$, and, although the precise intracellular molecular mechanisms of their actions are different, the net inhibitory effect in postsynaptic neurons is the same. This is further complicated by the fact that GABA receptors are composed of five protein subunits encoded by a family of genes. There are at least 16 different subunits that can interact with each other to form a $GABA_A$ receptor—six α subunits (α1–6), three β subunits (β1–3), three γ subunits (γ1–3) and one each of the $\delta, \epsilon, \vartheta$ and π subuits, and a similar complexity applies to $GABA_B$ receptors. Each and every one of these multiple receptors responds to GABA, although they have presumably evolved to provide slightly different responses in different circumstances and/or regions of the brain. For example, the $GABA_A$ receptor α1 subunit is the most abundant subunit in the brain and is present in 50 per cent of brain cells, but Purkinje cells in the cerebellum rely heavily on the α1 subunit as they do not express the other GABA α receptor subunits.

Most importantly, the presence of so many different GABA receptor subunits means that there is considerable redundancy—other receptors can do the same job (more or less) if one is inactivated, as the nerve cell can compensate using the large repertoire of other receptor subunits present in that cell. The genetic inactivation of one of the many GABA receptor subunit genes is therefore not necessarily lethal, and will have subtle effects that will specifically affect some brain cells more than others in different parts of the brain. Whilst all these defects will affect the circuitry that controls voluntary movement, each individual defect will have other manifestations. This might contribute to the observed heterogeneity of the movement disorder in ET.

It is important to emphasize that this proposed model of the causes of ET being a deficiency of GABA activity in a regulatory network in the brain is speculative. However, it is at least consistent with the several anti-tremor drugs that enhance inhibitory nerve cell activity, and it is consistent with the variability in the way ET manifests itself in different people. In addition, this hypothesis would also provide for the number of genetic targets required to explain both the observed genetic heterogeneity and the high incidence of ET worldwide.

Nevertheless, there is no direct evidence in humans that this model of the causes of ET is correct. For example, it could equally be caused by an excess of excitatory nerve cell activity. The functional and genetic complexity of other neurotransmitter receptors, including those that respond to dopamine, are comparable with that of the GABA receptors . Detailed investigations are required to understand fully the physiological consequences of a gene mutation or a particular phenotype such as ET in a living organism. Testing new drugs or surgical procedures on humans is always potentially dangerous and therefore has major moral and ethical implications. Anatomical analyses in humans rely largely on imaging, which has its limitations, or *post-mortem* examinations. The latter make it difficult to study disorders in their early stages, and the actual cause of death (old age in particular) is a potential confounding factor in interpreting post-mortem results.

Wherever possible, animal models are therefore used as they can be studied in exquisite detail using highly invasive techniques that would not be allowed in humans. Animals can also be used to test the safety and efficacy of new treatments, so if a new drug is toxic or has severe side-effects in the mouse, it is unlikely to be tried on humans. In the case of neurological disorders such as ET, and Alzheimer's and Parkinson's diseases, scientific research simply cannot be carried out in a test tube as a complex tissue such as the brain cannot be modelled in a test tube. Whilst animal experimentation should be kept to the minimum and rigorously regulated by law, scientific progress in understanding human disease currently still requires animal experimentation. ET is a heterogenous disorder that is complicated by environmental factors and the genetic heterogeneity of outbred human populations, so the results of human studies are often inconclusive. In contrast, the problems of genetic heterogeneity and environment do not apply in the laboratory mouse. Inbred mice offer a genetically homogenous background, and the environmental conditions in the animal house can be strictly controlled. Most importantly, the genetic make-up of the mice can be altered gene by gene using a *transgenic* approach.

A potentially very powerful approach to study the effects of a particular gene mutation in a live organism is to use genetic engineering to inactivate (knock-out) the gene in the laboratory mouse and see what happens in vivo. Mice have roughly the same number (30 000) of genes as humans, they have brains and a nervous system, and, in most cases, the same or very similar genes found in humans can be found in mice (gene homologues). In the first instance, one copy of the mouse gene is inactivated to give a heterozygous mouse ($+/-$; where $+$ is normal and $-$ is mutated), and then by selective breeding, a homozygous ($-/-$) knock-out transgenic mouse can be generated that cannot make the protein encoded by the targeted gene.

Animal models of human disease seldom arise by chance and have to be experimentally generated, but more often than not serendipity plays a major role and this is best illustrated by the genetically engineered ET mouse, which is the strongest evidence to support the proposed GABA receptor deficiency model in ET.

The GABA$_A$ α1 receptor subunit knock-out essential tremor mouse

Many psychoactive drugs target GABA receptors, and the large number of GABA$_A$ receptors composed of different protein subunits raised the possibility that different psychoactive drugs target different GABA$_A$ receptor subunit(s). To determine whether the GABA$_A$ receptor α1 subunit was targeted by different drugs, the gene encoding the α1 subunit was knocked out in transgenic mice to produce viable α1$^-$/α1$^-$ transgenic mice that were unable to make any α1 receptor subunit protein. The first reports of the pharmacological and electrophysiological responses of the α1$^-$/α1$^-$ knock-out mice do mention that the mice had an action tremor, but did not recognize that the tremor phenotype might be related to a human movement disorder. Eventually, the origin and type of tremor in the knock-out mice was investigated in depth and the investigators realized that it was an excellent model of the postural and kinetic tremor that is characteristic of ET.

To further validate the animal model, the investigators measured the frequency of the tremor and its response to the drugs routinely used to treat ET in humans. A 15–19 Hz tremor frequency was measured in the α1$^-$/α1$^-$ transgenic mice and, although this is significantly higher than the 4–12 Hz ET frequency observed in humans, this is most probably due to species-specific differences in the central nervous system and the smaller size of a mouse. Most significantly, the mouse tremor responded to the same drugs in the same way as the ET tremor in humans. Propranolol, primidone, alcohol (ethanol), gabapentin and an adenosine agonist (2-chloro-N^6-cyclopentyladenosine) all reduced the severity (amplitude but not frequency) of the mouse tremor as they do in human ET. Ethanol was the most potent of the drugs tested, and completely blocked the tremor in the transgenic mice at doses which were 'non-sedative'—in other words, the mice did not have to be completely drunk to stop shaking. Incidentally, this also showed that the anti-tremor effects of ethanol did not require GABA receptors that contain the α1 subunit.

The α1$^-$/α1$^-$ transgenic mice are quite normal other than having the tremor, so they must compensate for the absence of GABA$_A$ receptor α1 subunits in the brain and do this by increasing the expression of other GABA$_A$ receptor α subunits. This compensation changes the types of GABA$_A$ receptors in the brain compared with wild-type mice, and the response to psychoactive drugs that interact with GABA$_A$ receptors is therefore also changed. The available literature does not comment on the age of onset of the tremor in the transgenic mice, so it is unclear whether the action tremor is apparent as soon as the young mice (early onset) attempt voluntary movement. Similarly, it is not clear whether the tremor is progressive and increases in severity with age, although no doubt these studies are being performed.

The importance of the α1$^-$/α1$^-$ transgenic mouse cannot be underestimated. Human studies of ET have implicated the neuronal circuitry between cortex, the thalamus, the cerebellum, the basal ganglia, and the brainstem, and this circuitry can now be examined in detail in the transgenic mouse. For example, the Purkinje cells in the transgenic mouse were specifically examined because most of the GABA$_A$ receptors in Purkinje cells contain the α1 subunit and, unlike other parts of the brain, Purkinje cells do not seem to compensate for the absence of α1 subunits by expressing other α subunits. There was no evidence of α1$^-$/α1$^-$ cerebellar Purkinje cell death, but the cells were completely unresponsive to GABA.

The data are fascinating but should not be overinterpreted as the results are preliminary. Other cells in the brain including the thalamus express the GABA$_A$ receptor α1 subunit, so it is likely that the loss or impairment of GABA inhibition in other regions of the brain that control voluntary movement could be affected and contribute to the observed tremor, and it remains to be determined if loss of α1 subunits in any single brain area is sufficient to mimic human ET. Nevertheless, the α1$^-$/α1$^-$ transgenic mouse shows that a small deficiency in inhibitory GABA activity in the brain will cause a postural and kinetic tremor, and is consistent with the GABA-enhancing mode of action of the drugs currently used to treat ET. The mouse will be invaluable in further additional neurological studies and to test new drugs to treat ET.

Implications for the dominant mode of inheritance of essential tremor in humans

The postural and kinetic tremor observed in the homozygous $\alpha 1^-/\alpha 1^-$ transgenic mouse was not detected in the $\alpha 1^+/\alpha 1^-$ heterozygous mice who have one normal GABA$_A$ receptor $\alpha 1$ subunit gene. Genetically the $\alpha 1^-/\alpha 1^-$ mouse model of ET is therefore *recessive*—one normal copy of the gene is sufficient to prevent the tremor phenotype, and it is the complete absence of $\alpha 1$ receptor subunits that causes the action tremor. The *recessive* mode of inheritance in this mouse is in sharp contrast to the *dominant* mode of inheritance that has been inferred in the majority of cases of human familial ET (Chapter 5). This would appear to exclude mutations in GABA receptor subunit gene(s) as causal in human familial ET. However, the complex composition of GABA$_A$ receptors, together with our increasing understanding of how gene mutations can have a dominant effect despite the presence of a normal gene, suggest quite the contrary—certain types of mutation in GABA receptor subunit genes are precisely the sort of genetic alteration one would expect to be dominant. Gene mutations do not necessarily result in the complete loss of protein. If a mutant protein can still interact with other proteins, but the mutation affects the function of the protein complex as a whole, the effect of the mutation will be dominant as it is affecting the activity as a whole.

Consider a GABA$_A$ receptor composed of two $\alpha 1$ subunits, two $\beta 1$ subunits and one $\gamma 1$ subunit. Specific protein–protein interactions between the five subunits create the functional receptor that traverses the postsynaptic cell membrane to form a channel which can open when GABA binds (Fig. 6.3A). Imagine a mutation in one copy of the $\alpha 1$ subunit gene ($\alpha 1^M$) that allows the defective mutant $\alpha 1^M$ protein to interact with the other protein subunits, but introduces a change to the overall structure of the receptor near the channel and partially blocks it (Fig. 6.3B). Alternatively, the mutation might cause a structural change that makes the channel bigger and therefore more 'leaky' than normal (Fig. 6.3C).

A host of other possibilities can be envisaged where the one defective protein will disrupt the overall function of all five subunits in the protein complex that makes a functional receptor. Furthermore, the normal ($\alpha 1$) and mutant ($\alpha 1^M$) proteins are synthesized in roughly equal amounts as each is encoded by one gene in any one cell, so the number of normal $\alpha 1$ or mutant $\alpha 1^M$ protein subunits in any one GABA$_A$ receptor is a matter of chance during receptor assembly. The receptor could contain zero, one or two mutant $\alpha 1^M$ or normal $\alpha 1$ proteins (Fig. 6.3). However, as the presence of one or two $\alpha 1^M$ proteins in the receptor complex is sufficient to disrupt normal receptor function, the single gene mutation will disrupt two out of

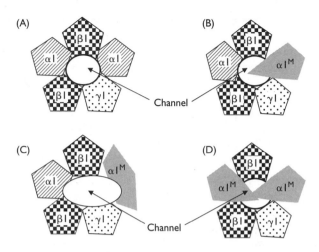

Figure 6.3 Dominant gene mutations and the GABA$_A$ receptor-gated ion channel. (A) Schematic representation of a normal GABA$_A$ receptor complex composed of five proteins (two α1, two β1 and one γ). The proteins form a channel on the surface of the postsynaptic cell when bound by GABA neurotransmitter to allow direct communication between the inside and outside of the cell . The α1 protein is encoded by the α1 gene. In this hypothetical scenario, an α1 receptor gene mutation (α1^M) alters the structure and/or function of the receptor protein although it can still interact with the other four proteins in the receptor complex, including the normal α1 proteins as most affected individuals also inherit a normal gene (α1/α1^M) and make both proteins in similar amounts. As both normal and mutant proteins are made in the same cell, all four combinations of receptor will be assembled. Three possible effects can be considered. (B) Both normal (α1) and abnormal (α1^M) protein can be found in the same receptor complex. The α1^M protein partially blocks the gated ion channel. (C) The α1^M protein might change the shape and size of the channel to make it leaky. (D) Two α1^M proteins in a receptor might fully block the channel. Although one-third of the receptors will be normal (A), two-thirds will be abnormal (B–D) to give a dominant genetic trait in a heterozygous (α1/α1^M) individual.

three (66 per cent) of all GABA$_A$ receptors assembled by the cell. If the altered activities of the leaky (Fig. 6.3C) or blocked (Fig. 6.3D) channels also disrupt the initiation and/or propagation of the desired GABA inhibitory signal, then the single gene mutation will indeed overwhelm the function of the remaining 33 per cent of normal receptors—the gene mutation is thus *dominant*. To all intents and purposes, the normal protein is inactivated by the dominant mutant protein, resulting in the absence of normal protein as would be found in a recessive genetic disorder and exemplified in $\alpha1^-/\alpha1^-$ knock-out transgenic mice.

The general principle that many dominant mutations do not affect protein–protein interactions, but affect the overall function of multimeric protein complexes which contain the mutant proteins, is a useful reminder that protein products encoded by genes do not act in isolation within a cell. The proteins are interacting with themselves and with other proteins, and it is these specific interactions that confer the desired biochemical activity on the protein complex(es). Mutation of any one of the protein subunits in a complex can have a profound *dominant* effect on the whole.

Conclusions

The $GABA_A$ $\alpha1$ receptor subunit knock-out mouse represents the most significant and interesting ET experimental result in recent years. It will fundamentally change current thinking about the possible causes of ET. Speculation about the specific role of different regions of the brain in ET will be superseded by the knowledge that a general deficit of inhibitory neuronal activity in the brain can result in ET-like symptoms and is obviously consistent with the fact that GABA agonists are used to treat the ET tremor in the clinic. The ET-causing inhibitory activity deficit may be restricted to specific neurons or regions of the brain, but the local effects of this deficit can now be examined in specific regions of the mouse brain if appropriate. In addition to providing an invaluable experimental model for further neurological studies, the ET mouse provides a concrete intellectual platform that will transform our understanding of ET and thus both stimulate and accelerate progress in both academia and the clinic. In future, other GABA receptor subunit genes will be knocked out in the mouse to provide further evidence that distinct genetic defects can cause ET. As such, the mouse discovery is probably as important to ET as the original discovery of tremor-related neuronal activity in the thalamus.

7 The future: what are the prospects of a cure for essential tremor?

Looking into the not so distant future, we can imagine a time when molecular biologists and medical geneticists have identified the defective gene(s) and neurologists have identified how that defect leads to the periodic ET-related neuronal firing that causes ET. They may also identify the precise anatomical position and physiological properties of the defective nerve cells that cause ET. Armed with this information, it should be possible to develop a cure for ET.

The word 'cure' implies that following a course or one-off treatment, an individual will be permanently free of ET. Ever since it was formally demonstrated that specific gene mutations cause specific disorders, logic has dictated that the disorder would be cured if the gene defect could be repaired, or the defective gene replaced by a functional normal copy. However, the main difficulty is how to get the normal gene into all the affected cells that cause ET. Furthermore, it is necessary to ensure that the normal gene is expressed (makes protein) in the right amounts at the right time in the right cells, and ensure above all else that this form of genetic manipulation has no unwanted side effects.

An alternative approach, which avoids the technically difficult task of repairing or replacing one gene in many cells, is to replace the faulty cells with normal (or engineered) cells. 'Normal' cells are placed where they are needed and will do the job the resident mutant or damaged cells are unable to perform. In ET, this would be equivalent to a mini brain transplant, as nerve cells would be transplanted into the affected region of the brain to take over and stop the tremor-related neuronal activity. However, there are several steps to success: first, the cells need to be transplanted into the correct region of the brain, whilst minimizing further, and potentially more serious, brain damage with the procedure. Second, the transplanted cells must not elicit an immune response from the host or they will be rejected—rejection is the single most serious risk in all organ transplants. Third, the transplanted cells must do exactly what is required in the brain—no more or less—as any deviation from the desired programme could lead to the cells misbehaving in a critical part of the brain with unfortunate and unpredictable side effects. Finally, the transplanted cells must be able to survive in the host brain for life, and must therefore be able to divide in a controlled manner and respond to the physiological signals within the brain's environment. The cells that are most promising for therapeutic transplantation are called '*stem cells*'. Stem cell research, which is currently perhaps one of the most controversial subjects in the life sciences, nevertheless has enormous clinical potential as a treatment known as '*stem cell therapy*'.

Although gene therapy and stem cell therapy have been tried out on human beings, and some of these trials will be mentioned, major problems have been encountered. Finding solutions to these problems is the subject of active research worldwide, and both approaches are being developed and perfected in numerous laboratories. However, this effort has relied to a large extent on animal experimentation, so an overview of some of the more promising results will be provided.

Gene therapy

A single diploid cell is a tiny more or less self-contained entity that contains 60 000 genes encoded by a lot of DNA (a string of 6 000 000 000 As, Ts, Cs and Gs). Suppose all the cells in a person with ET have a mutation in one gene that is directly responsible for the ET. The gene corresponds to about 0.0005 per cent of the DNA in every brain cell, and the mutation is a single C to G letter change within the gene that changes the function of the protein encoded (made from that gene). The logistics of repairing this single base mutation in each and every one of the cells that cause the tremor are daunting. The DNA mechanic has to find that one specific base in the cell's DNA, and then change that one incorrect G back to a C. As all DNA is a long string of As, Ts, Cs and Gs, it is very difficult to envisage a repair mechanism that can identify the one incorrect G that is causing the problem, and this process has to be carried out in hundreds if not thousands of other cells in the living brain.

A simpler approach is to put a normal functioning copy of the abnormal gene back into the cells that cause the shaking—the defective copy already present in the cell can be ignored as the functionally normal gene will be used to make working protein that will stop tremor irrespective of what the defective gene is or is not doing. However, there are several problems with the replacement approach to gene therapy:

- The gene has to be delivered to all the cells in a living brain.
- Assuming the delivery problem is solved, the gene has to be stable in the recipient cells so that it is passed on (replicated) if and when those cells divide.

- Assuming a stable copy of the gene can be delivered to the cells, it must be switched on (expressed) so that normal functioning protein can be made by the recipient cells.

- The genetic engineering process must not have any unwanted effects on the recipient cells.

The most efficient way of delivering DNA into a cell is to use viruses, as they have evolved to introduce their genetic material into a host cell. The virus then highjacks the cellular machinery to make more viruses which then infect more cells—this usually kills the infected host cells. If uncontrolled, this will also kill the infected organism, and incidentally kill the virus as well. So it represents a serious evolutionary problem to the virus—its success will kill it. The virus would soon become extinct. Viruses have therefore evolved a second more insidious strategy—rather than making more viruses and killing the cell, the viral genetic information is occasionally integrated into the cellular DNA where it remains stable and dormant—undetected by the body's immune defence mechanisms. It can then re-awaken at some future time and the whole process is then repeated. The success of a virus depends on its ability to make more viruses and infect other people, without killing the infected individual before it has had a chance to procreate.

One example that illustrates both the importance of the immune system and the insidious ways viruses work is the human immunodeficiency virus (HIV). HIV specifically infects and kills cells (T cells) that are absolutely required to mount an immune response against viruses (including HIV itself) and other infectious agents. As the HIV virus kills these essential T cells, the immune system is severely damaged, and the body cannot defend itself. Infected individuals are immune deficient and therefore highly susceptible to opportunistic infections—hence AIDS (acquired immune deficiency syndrome). It takes a long time for the HIV to kill the infected individual; HIV-positive individuals can be quite healthy for many years before the first symptoms become apparent. The unaware host may infect other individuals, enabling viruses to spread and exploit the long latency to survive.

Viruses can be engineered so that they are not infectious and thus do not generate more viruses or kill the infected person's cells. Similarly, the desired gene can be engineered into the viral DNA so that it is transported to the cells by the disabled virus, where it is injected into the cells. The viral (and gene) DNA will then integrate into the cell's own (cellular) DNA. This in principle achieves all the requirements for an efficient delivery system.

One typical example where gene therapy should have worked but did not is cystic fibrosis (CF), which is caused by a mutation in a particular gene

(CFTR). The most life-threatening problem (which is extremely unpleasant for the patient) occurs in the lungs, which become blocked by the production of thick mucus. The engineered virus and a normal copy of the CFTR gene can easily be delivered to all the cells in the lung in the form of an aerosol that is inhaled by the patient—all the lung cells are exposed to the normal gene in one breath. Unfortunately, trials using this approach showed that, although the gene was effectively taken up by many of the lung cells, they did not switch on the inhaled gene, very little normal CFTR protein was made, and there was no significant therapeutic benefit.

To get around the problem of keeping the gene switched on, a patient's cells can be infected in the test tube and the few cells that do express the normal gene can be grown in quantity, purified, and then transplanted back into the patient. As will be described in a little more detail below, the cells that are most amenable to growing in the laboratory and being genetically modified are the stem cells. The best characterized stem cells are the bone marrow cells responsible for making all our blood cells, so gene therapy has also been targeted at blood disorders. It is a relatively simple procedure to aspirate some bone marrow from a patient, infect the cells in a test tube, select those cells that are expressing reasonable amounts of the therapeutic gene, and then put the cells back into the patient. Moderate successes have been reported using this approach, but it is well known that viruses can cause cancer. This unfortunate side effect that was predicted by many experts has been found.

One blood cell disorder that was treated by the viral transfer of the normal gene into bone marrow cells was the X-linked severe combined immunodeficiency disease (X-SCID). X-SCID is also known as the 'bubble-baby syndrome'—the children literally have no immune defence and are therefore brought up in the sterile environment of a plastic isolation chamber (the bubble) to prevent life-threatening infections. The defective X-SCID gene has been identified, and the normal gene engineered into a virus. This virus was then used to infect the patients' bone marrow cells, which were then transplanted back into affected children. The clinical trials began in Paris in 1999, and nine out of 11 children showed tremendous improvements in their immune system and were able to live relatively normal lives outside their bubbles. Unfortunately, two of the 11 boys developed leukaemia (a bone marrow cell cancer) 3 years later. The reason for this was that the virus used for gene therapy had indeed gone into the cellular DNA (integrated) next to a cancer-causing gene (*oncogene*). There are a number of technical ways of reducing this kind of risk, but for now gene therapy trials have either been put on hold or told to proceed with extreme caution.

At least two cases of leukaemia and one death have so far been reported in clinical gene therapy trials. Playing with cellular DNA will always carry this risk. However, the therapeutic benefits in the X-SCID patients were spectacular but, as usual, there is a fine balance between benefit and risk—unfortunately, a 20 per cent risk of leukaemia is not insignificant, and this excessive risk has to be reduced before this gene therapy approach can become established in the clinic.

Stem cells

Day-to-day existence causes a lot of damage to cells in many tissues. The damaged/dead cells are continually replaced so that the self-renewing cellular processes are to a certain extent immortal as they last a lifetime. There are several tissues in the body that suffer particularly severe wear and tear and have to be continually replenished/repaired as cells die off. The most obvious examples are listed below.

- The skin: the surface of the skin is continually being sloughed off due to damage caused by day-to-day wear and tear or injury—one obvious manifestation of dead skin falling away is dandruff. Skin has the inherent ability to self-renew and will last for a lifetime. Although our skin will undoubtedly age (wrinkles, etc.), we will never run out of skin.

- The gut: the cells in the gut which are responsible for digesting our food and absorbing the nutrients into the bloodstream suffer considerably from the highly physical process involved in digestion in a potentially toxic environment. Like the skin, the key cells in the gut are continually being sloughed off and replaced.

- Bone marrow: we need red blood cells in the blood to carry oxygen from the lungs to all the tissues, and to carry carbon dioxide from the tissues back to the lungs. As a result of travelling around the body in the bloodstream and being squeezed through tiny blood vessels (capillaries) to reach all the cells throughout the body, the red blood cells inevitably get damaged and are destroyed (actually recycled). Each and every red blood cell has to be replaced every 2–3 weeks, and roughly 1 000 000 000 000 red blood cells have to be made every day in a typical adult human.

The cells that are able to maintain tissues for life are called *stem cells*, and they have two key properties:

Self-renewal: they are able to 'self-renew'—they will divide to produce two identical copies of themselves. One copy can then go on to become a more mature cell that is eventually lost through wear and tear, whilst the other maintains its stem cell properties. The total number of stem cells therefore remains relatively constant throughout adult life, despite the production of huge numbers of daughter cells that are used to replace high-turnover cells in tissues.

Differentiation: in addition to red blood cells, blood contains a number of other specialized cells that are needed to fight infection and produce platelets for blood clotting. These highly specialized cells are all derived from the same stem cell in the bone marrow. The stem cells can therefore become any one of these specialized cells in a process called *differentiation*. The production of mature blood cells by the bone marrow stem cells is a highly regulated process and is well able to respond to stress to increase the numbers of particular cells in the blood. For example, blood loss requires more red blood cells (*erythrocytes*) to compensate for the reduced oxygen-carrying capacity of the blood. The body responds by producing a hormone (*erythropoietin*; *Epo*) that will specifically stimulate the production of more red blood cells by the bone marrow, and restore the oxygen-carrying capacity of the blood. Stem cells can thus be persuaded to differentiate into different cells by giving them the appropriate growth factor signal.

Similar processes occur in the skin (and intestine). The basal layer of the skin contains the stem cells which self-renew and differentiate. The differentiating cells are pushed upwards through the various layers of the skin, and as they move upwards they become harder until they reach the surface of the skin to provide the hard protective layer of dead cells and replace previous cells that had been sloughed off through day-to-day wear and tear.

It has recently become apparent that almost every tissue in the living body has stem cells. Even more surprising is that a bone marrow stem cell can actually become a brain cell, or a muscle cell, so a large number of differentiation options are open to a stem cell, and this has transformed our understanding of human cellular biology. The potential clinical applications of stem cell therapy are huge, as any tissue damage/defect can in principle be repaired by transplanting stem cells into that tissue. Most significantly, stem cells can be grown in the laboratory, and can be genetically engineered before being transplanted back into a recipient.

The stem cell controversy

The ultimate stem cell is the fertilized egg! A single fertilized egg can divide and differentiate to generate every specialized cell in the body, including other stem cells. Studies in mice first demonstrated that stem cells could be isolated from pre-implantation embryos (*blastocysts*) and grown indefinitely in the laboratory. These are known as embryonal stem (ES) cells. ES cells can then be injected back into an early embryo which in turn can be placed back in to a pseudo-pregnant female, and the embryo will develop into a viable mouse.

The mouse will have some cells derived from the original recipient embryo but will also have cells derived from the donor ES cells that were injected into it. In experimental animals, further selective breeding can yield a mouse that is completely composed of cells derived from the donor ES cells. Furthermore, the ES cells can be genetically modified to inactivate a particular gene (*knock-out*) or to produce a specific protein (*knock-in*) before being transplanted into an embryo. Genetically engineered organisms are called 'transgenic' (see also Chapter 6).

Human ES cells can also be grown in the laboratory, so humans can in principle be genetically modified. Most people are fully aware of the complex ethical/moral problems this raises. Auguments that it goes against the will of God/nature, and the prospect of genetically engineered superhumans taking over the world and demoting ordinary mortals to a biological underclass has been fully, but inaccurately, aired in the media. As most desirable human phenotypes (e.g. intelligence) are determined by a large number of genes which are in turn greatly influenced by the environment (nature versus nurture), it is extremely unlikely that the genetic modification of any one single gene will produce a significant change in the desired phenotype (intelligence) of the offspring.

ES cells, by definition, have to be isolated from a developing embryo, and this raises the thorny moral/ethical issue of when a collection of cells becomes a 'human being'. Early embryos can be generated by *in vitro* fertilization in the laboratory, or obtained from abortions, but to 'pro-life' campaigners this is unacceptable. Pro-life campaigners have put the US Government under enormous pressure to halt or restrict the research into ES cell biology. Severe restrictions have been imposed on ES cell research in the USA, notwithstanding intense pressure from celebrities (including Nancy Reagan, Michael J. Fox and Mohammed Ali) to allow this type of research to be carried out, as it offers the potential of cures for Alzheimer's and Parkinson's diseases, and for paralysis due to damage to the spinal cord. European and Asian countries tend to be more relaxed about human ES cell research.

The use of stem cells in transplantations to repair damaged or defective tissues still has the problem of rejection by the recipient's immune system. ES cells, like other organs, have to be matched for immune compatability prior to transplantation, but, in principle, a large bank of different ES cells could be kept in the laboratory so that at least one ES cell would match each and every recipient. Alternatively, as large numbers of stem cells have been found in the blood of the umbilical cord immediately after birth, these stem cells could be harvested and stored indefinitely. Every individual would thus have his or her own store of stem cells—there would be no problem with rejection. The frozen cells could be used later in life to repair a damaged tissue, or could be genetically engineered before being transplanted back into the recipient to repair the defect. This would only be of any use to people born after the introduction of an umbilical cord stem cell banking system.

It is reasonable to assume that the technical problems of using stem cells in therapies can be overcome. The moral and ethical issues need to be addressed by society as a whole. Perhaps when stem cells have been used to treat particularly nasty diseases successfully, and people are reassured that the stem cells will not/cannot be used to produce an engineered super-race, public opinion might be swayed.

Stem cell therapy in neurodegenerative disorders

Neural stem cells and Parkinson's disease

The discovery that most tissues (including the brain) have their own stem cells raises the exciting prospect of using stem cells to repair damaged tissues in progressive neurodegenerative disorders. Parkinson's disease is a prime candidate for stem cell therapy, as damaged cells in particular regions of the brain can, in principle, be replaced by healthy brain cells to cure, reduce or halt the progression of the disease, and improve function. In Parkinson's disease, the progressive degeneration (death) of specific nerve cells that use the excitatory neurotransmitter dopamine in an area of the brain called the substantia nigra pars compacta (SNc) provides a good situation to test the simple concept that cells can be transplanted into the brain and either repair or replace damaged cells and thus improve dopamine production.

The developing fetal brain is an excellent source of neurons, which have already been primed to become brain cells, are 'young and healthy', and have not fully established the interneuronal connections found in the adult brain. Although they are not stem cells, they have been transplanted into the brains of patients with Parkinson's disease. These cells have been shown to survive for as long as 10 years, make apparently normal connections with other neurons, and are functionally integrated into the neuronal circuitry of the brain. Furthermore, dopamine production can be increased and the initiation of movement is improved. In some patients, modest to good benefits have been reported, although the ongoing destruction of the patient's own dopamine-producing cells continues. However, up to 15 per cent of Parkinson's patients who received fetal neural cells subsequently suffered from 'runaway dyskinesias' (out of control involuntary movements). In Parkinson's disease, dyskinesias are normally seen in response to prolonged treatment and in particular to overdosage with dopaminergic drugs. However, in patients who have received fetal transplants, the 'runaway dyskinesias' occur even when no dopaminergic treatment is administered. The mechanisms underlying these runaway dyskinesias are poorly understood, but may include incomplete engraftment in the damaged region of the brain, overproduction of dopamine by the transplanted cells, or chronic inflammation and immune responses around the grafted cells (rejection). Little clinical benefit would be achieved in more severely disabled patients where the neurodegeneration is particularly advanced.

Whilst fetal cell engraftment is very promising, it is fraught with logistic, ethical and moral problems. The only source of these cells is from freshly aborted fetuses, and this is even more controversial than utilizing ES cells. Even though fetal cell grafting has been performed for Parkinson's disease for well over a decade, relatively few procedures of this type have actually been done and the method is still considered to be experimental.

Thus in the absence of a steady supply of fetal neural cells, the easiest solution is to grow the cells in the laboratory—an infinite number of cells can be grown (if necessary in large industrial vats). The cells are perceived by the general public as much less 'human' than an aborted fetus, and are normally incapable of generating a whole viable organism. However, fetal nerve cells will not grow in the test-tube (*in vitro*). The only type of cells that can be grown indefinitely *in vitro*, and which have the potential to become dopamine-producing neurons, are (neural) stem cells. Neural stem cells can be transplanted back into a brain where they will settle in, differentiate and become part of the working brain, but the source of neural stem cells is also controversial as the fetus is again the richest source. Stem cells from other tissues (bone marrow in particular) are highly 'plastic' and can be persuaded to differentiate into neural cells, so the use of stem cells from the patient's own body avoids the rejection and ethical problems. However, such stem cell transplantations carry a high risk (up to 20 per cent) that some of the stem cells will carry on growing without differentiation and produce a tumour (teratoma). This risk decreases significantly if the cells are differentiated *in vitro* prior to transplantation, so it is clearly safer to use committed neural stem cells.

ES cells can be persuaded to differentiate specifically into a variety of progenitor and mature neural cells *in vitro* using chemical and biological agents. In principle, once the cells are committed to become neural cells, or sufficient numbers of cells are fully differentiated (e.g. dopamine-producing cells for Parkinson's disease), they can be transplanted back into the damaged area of the brain where they would repair the damage. This approach has been successfully attempted in the brain and spinal cord of experimental rodents, where they have engrafted and differentiated into neurons and glial cells. There is no doubt that ES cells have the potential to rebuild the nervous system in a clinical context, but for the moment they have to be primed to become brain cells before transplantation. The efficiency of the chemical and biological agents that are used to induce neural differentiation is not 100 per cent, so whilst they may be highly enriched for neural progenitor cells, they are not pure, raising the possibility of complications after transplantation.

Damage in the brain produces signals that will stimulate repair by resident neural stem cells. However, in the case of severe damage, the small numbers of resident stem cells in the adult brain are unable to repair that damage. An alternative approach is to try and stimulate that small number of resident neural stem cells in the brain of the affected adult individual to proliferate and differentiate to repair or replace damaged nerve cells. The key growth factor required for the growth of neural stem cells is glial cell line-derived neurotrophic factor (GDNF). Whilst endogenous neural stem cells may not have the ability to prevent or repair neurological damage on their own, they might if they received a sufficiently strong (e.g. GDNF) signal that would kick-start their proliferation so they would carry out the repair/replacement themselves. However, the blood–brain barrier prevents GDNF being delivered to the brain by either oral or intravenous administration. Because transplanted neural stem cells will engraft into the brain, transplanting stem cells that have been engineered in the laboratory to produce GDNF (or any other growth factor) is an alternative therapeutic approach. The transplanted cells do not have to do much—they just have to survive and produce a steady supply of GDNF in the brain that will mobilize and stimulate the endogenous stem cells into action and repair the damage. In principle, this could be applied to any tissue in the body which has resident stem cells that can be stimulated by specific growth factors, and has led to the concept of a stem cell-mediated 'mini-pump' which has also been nicknamed the 'fountain of youth' as it could replace tissues lost during the normal ageing process.

The key question that remains is whether these cells have any clinical benefit. Most of the evidence comes from animal experiments, and a few should be considered. One has to bear in mind that animal models may not necessarily fully represent the human disease, and that different strategies may be required depending on whether the aim is to repair existing nerve cells, to replace damaged nerve cells or to correct a biochemical imbalance.

Animal models in stem cell therapy

Experimenting with mice is important because a number of variables that will potentially determine the effectiveness of the putative therapy to repair a very specific defect can be examined carefully in the controlled environment of the laboratory. How many stem cells? Where is the best place to implant them? What are the side effects? There is always a risk as new therapies are developed and perfected, so using animals as models is the only available option. These and others are key questions that have to be answered before the procedure can be tried out in humans.

In addition to naturally occurring mouse mutants such as the Shiverer (*Shi*) mouse, genetic engineers can mutate specific genes in the mouse in order to create an experimental transgenic model of any one particular disorder. There are ET mice ($GABA_A\alpha1$ receptor gene mutations; Chapter 6), Parkinson's disease mice (parkin gene mutations), and Huntington's disease (HD gene mutations) mice. Alternatively, researchers can use surgical lesions or specific poisons to kill or damage specific brain or spinal cord cells, and thus mimic particular human disorders.

Gene and stem cell therapies have been tried on some of these (and many other) mouse models with some success. However, they have also identified potential problems. The ongoing research in animal models is essential as it will allow scientists to try out different strategies and different cells, and thus perfect, as far as possible, the techniques prior to clinical trials in humans.

Gene and stem cell therapy in essential tremor

The fundamental problem in ET is that compared with the many degenerative neurological disorders, the exact problem in ET is unknown. Stem cell therapy for ET cannot even be considered an option until the precise defect has been identified, and there is currently no specific neurological target to aim for. Scientists are currently, to all intents and purposes, blind, although this will hopefully change with time. In the future, scientists may try to engineer the stem cells prior to transplantation so that they produce, for example, GABA (or GABA agonists), as there is some evidence that this might help ET if the correct site(s) for implantation could be found.

Currently, the understanding of ET is poor compared with other movement disorders—for example Parkinson's and Huntington's diseases. Whilst our understanding of ET may be lagging behind, there is every reason to believe that advances in the understanding of other neurological disorders will pave the way for the swift application of new technologies to ET. ET may be the poor and neglected relation in movement disorders, but it will ultimately benefit from the scientific and clinical experience gained from the treatment of the neurodegenerative movement disorders.

Perhaps in the future, science will show that ET is caused by a simple change in certain receptors involved in the circuits that control voluntary movement.

8 Glossary

Accelerometer: a small piezo-electric device that is attached to the back of the patient's hand with tape. It is commonly used to record tremor, and works by measuring the acceleration and deceleration movements of the patient's hand caused by tremor in m/s/s.

Acetylcholine (ACh): excitatory neurotransmitter, used in the communication between nerve cells and muscle. Blocked by *curare*.

Action tremor: tremor that occurs during any voluntary action.

Adenosine: used to make DNA, but also used as an inhibitory *neuromodulator* of nerve cell activity.

Adrenaline: see epinephrine.

β-Adrenergic: cells that respond to noradrenaline or epinephrine.

Agonist: promotes an effect.

Allodynia: hypersensitivity to pain.

Antagonist: inhibits or opposes an effect.

Anxiogenic: promotes anxiety.

Anxiolytic: reduces anxiety.

Autonomic nervous system: nervous system responsible for the automatic visceral 'rest and digest' and 'fight or flight' responses of the body.

Axon: long process of a nerve cell used to transmit electrical signals over long distances.

Barbiturate: phenobarbital—hypnotic. See *primidone*

Benzodiazepines: chlordiazepoxide (Librium) and diazepam (Valium) are two of the most common examples—anti-anxiety and muscle-relaxing drugs. GABA agonists.

Beta-blocker: β-adrenergic blocker—blocks the activity of noradrenaline and epinephrine predominantly in the autonomic nervous system. See *propranolol.*

Bilateral tremor: tremor occurs on both sides of the body (both arms, hands, etc.).

Botulinum toxin: a toxin (poison) that blocks the release of acetylcholine neurotransmitter, leading to muscle paralysis.

Bradykinesia: a reduced speed of voluntary movement; slowness of movement typically seen in Parkinson's disease, and not essential tremor.

Cannabis: a group of psychoactive compounds produced from the *Cannabis sativa* plant. Also called marijuana and hemp. See *THC*.

Catalepsy: a frozen motionless rigid state.

Cerebellum: area of the brain located at the back of the skull involved in controlling and fine tuning voluntary movement.

Computerized tomography (CT): a CT scan involves the transmission of a thin beam of X-rays through the part of the body being examined. The attenuated X-rays are recorded and reflect the electron density of the tissue through which they have passed. This process is repeated from various angles and at small intervals (slices). A computer then reconstructs all the X-ray images to form a two- or three-dimensional picture.

Concordance: a measure of the frequency with which both members of monozygotic and dizygotic twin pairs share the same genetic and phenotypic trait.

Curare (D-tubocurarine): isolated from the bark of a South American tree (*Strychnos toxifera*) and used as an arrow poison. Potent blocker of acetylcholine receptors.

Delerium tremens: trembling and hallucinations brought on by chronic alcoholism.

Dementia: a clinical syndrome characterized by progressive memory decline and impairment of at least one other cognitive domain.

Dendrite: the part of a postsynaptic cell that receives the signal that originated in the presynaptic cell.

Differentiation: the process that converts an unspecialized stem or progenitor cell into a mature highly specialized cell.

Diploid: a cell that has two copies of the genome and pairs of each of the non-sex chromosomes: one copy inherited from the mother and one from the father.

Dizygotic twins: non-identical twins born as a consequence of the chance fertilization of two different eggs by two different sperm at the same time. Genetically equivalent to any other two siblings.

DNA: deoxyribonucleic acid. A double helix composed of two antiparallel helical sugar-phosphate backbones, and with bases attached to the sugar residues such that the interaction between complementary bases (A:T and G:C) specifically stabilize the two strands. A three letter code in a *gene* encodes one amino acid in a protein.

Dominant: describes a mode of inheritance where the inheritance of one gene is sufficient to cause the phenotype. Heterozygotes ($+/-$) are affected, and typically affected family members are found in every generation.

Dopamine: excitatory neurotransmitter, binds to *dopaminergic* nerve cells.

Dopamine transporter (DAT): an active transport pump that clears dopamine from the synaptic cleft. DAT is located to in the membranes of the axons and dendrites of the dopamine-containing neurons in the nigrostriatal region of the brain.

Dysarthria: difficulty speaking.

Dyskinesia: involuntary movement, most commonly seen in Parkinson's disease after long-term exposure to levodopa, or in schizophrenia after long-term treatment with dopamine receptor-blocking drugs.

Dysmetria: the tendency for the patient's hand to under- or overshoot or miss a target when attempting to touch it. See *intention tremor*.

Dystonia: co-contraction of agonist and antagonist muscles leading to abnormal postures, slow involuntary movements and pain.

Efferent neurons: neurons connecting the brain to the spinal cord.

Electromyography (EMG): measurement of electrical activity in muscles either using electrodes placed on the skin above the muscle (surface EMG) or using a needle inserted into the muscle.

Endocannabinoids: chemicals produced by the brain that bind to the same receptor and have the same effect as *THC* in *cannabis*.

Epinephrine (adrenaline): produced by the adrenal gland in response to stress. Triggered by the hypothalamus, it is involved in the 'fight or flight' response to a threat

Excitatory: fascilitates, stimulates.

Functional magnetic resonance imaging (fMRI): fMRI is a non-invasive imaging technique (scanner) that exploits the different magnetic properties of blood carrying oxygen (diamagnetic) and blood that has been depleted of oxygen (paramagnetic). The local increase in energy requirements during neuronal firing in the brain requires an increase in oxygen which is delivered by an increase in the local oxygenated blood flow (the *haemodynamic response*). The magnitude of change in MRI signal intensity is used as an indirect measure of changes in neuronal activity (see also MRI).

GABA: γ-aminobutyric acid. An inhibitory neurotransmitter.

Gabapentin (neurotonin): structurally and functionally very similar to the inhibitory GABA neurotransmitter. Mainly used as an anti-convulsant in the treatment of epilepsy but can be used to treat essential tremor.

Gene: the DNA sequence required to encode a specific protein. Includes regulatory elements that ensure the particular protein is made in the right amount in the right cell(s) at the right time. The fundamental unit of heredity.

Genotype: the specific genetic constitution of an organism. In ET this would be homozygous for the normal gene (ET^+/ET^+), or either heterozygous (ET^+/ET^-) or (rarely) homozygous (ET^-/ET^-) for the mutant gene.

Germline: collective name for the eggs and sperm used in reproduction.

Glial cells: Greek name for glue. These cells play a key role in protecting, supporting, and nourishing neurons. *Oligodendrocytes* and *Schwann* cells are glial cells that generate the insulating myelin sheath around axons in the central and peripheral nervous systems, respectively. Other glial cells (*astrocytes*; star shaped) are involved in generating the impermeable and protective blood–brain barrier.

Glial-derived neurotrophic factor (GDNF): a growth factor produced by glial cells that stimulates the proliferation of neural stem cells.

Glycine: an amino acid. Also used as an inhibitory neurotransmitter.

Glutamate: excitatory neurotransmitter.

Hemiparesis: weakness down one side of the body, typically affecting one half of the face, the arm, and leg.

Haploid: contains only one copy of the genome (cf. *diploid*).

Heritability: a measure of how much the variation in *a phenotype* is due to genetics. A low heritability score implicates environmental factors.

Hertz (Hz): the frequency of an oscillating or periodic wave 1 Hz = 1 cycle per second.

Heterozygous: carrying one normal and one mutant gene ($+/-$).

Homologues: members of a chromosome pair in a diploid cell, e.g. chromosome 2.

Homozygous: carrying two copies of a normal $(+/+)$ or mutant $(-/-)$ gene.

Hyperkinetic: too much involuntary movement (e.g. essential tremor).

Hypokinetic: too little movement (e.g. Parkinson's disease).

Inhibitory: suppresses, inhibits.

Intention tremor: this is a type of tremor in which the amplitude of the tremor increases towards the end of a visually guided movement of the arm towards a target (e.g. trying to touch a particular point on a touch-screen computer). This type of tremor may be associated with impairments of co-ordination, for example with a tendency to overshoot the target during movement (see dysmetria).

Kinetic tremor: tremor occurring during any voluntary movement.

Levodopa (L-DOPA; L-dihydroxyphenylalanine): dopamine precursor, used in drug replacement therapy in Parkinson's disease.

Micrographia: small writing. Micrographia is typically exhibited by Parkinson's disease sufferers.

Magnetic resonance imaging (MRI): the concentration and magnetic characteristics of certain atoms in the body can be detected by applying a strong magnetic field and a radio signal perpendicular to the magnetic field in order to make the nuclei spin coherently together (resonate). When the applied radio signal is stopped, the nuclei begin to dephase and a radio signal is emitted from the nuclei within the atoms. This is converted to an image by projection onto a matrix and assigned levels of grey. In general, MRI has a greater sensitivity to pathological change than CT.

Meiosis: the process of generating haploid gametes (eggs and sperm) from a diploid precursor stem cell. Involves one round of DNA synthesis followed by two rounds of cell division. An obligatory recombination event between chromosome homologues is required.

Meiotic recombination: exchange of genetic information between newly replicated chromosome homologues.

Monozygotic twins: identical twins. The fertilization of one egg by one sperm sometimes leads to the production of two genetically identical offspring.

Myelin sheath: insulation around neuronal axons provided by glial cells.

Neuromodulator: a molecule that influences synaptic transmission without itself being a neurotransmitter (see *adenosine*).

Neuron: nerve cell.

Neuropathology: the study of the pathology (abnormalitites in the tissues) of the nervous system.

Neuropathy: a neurological disorder, which has a multitude of causes, in which the peripheral nerves are damaged.

Neurotransmitter: chemical messenger that is secreted by a presynaptic cell, crosses the synapse, and binds a receptor on the postsynaptic cell.

Nodes of Ranvier: short gaps in the myelin sheath insulation of axons used to regenerate the electrical impulse as it travels.

Oncogene: a mutated gene capable of causing cancer.

Paraesthesia: abnormal sensation (e.g. burning or tickling) on the surface of the body.

Penetrance: the probability that a (disease) phenotype will appear when a disease-related genotype has been inherited. Often not 100 per cent.

Phenotype: the genetically controlled, observable properties of an organism or person.

Placebo: an inactive but harmless preparation given at random to patients in clinical trials to act as controls for the new drug being trialled.

Polymorphism: the occurrence of two or more genotypes in a population. A DNA sequence difference between each of the two copies of a gene that does not necessarily have a phenotypic effect.

Positron emission tomography (PET): uses a short-lived radioactive tracer which decays by emitting a positron. The chemical is injected into the living subject and accumulates in the target tissue. The short-lived isotope decays, emitting a positron which is detected by a scanner. In neurology, radioactive oxygen (^{15}O) or glucose are often used as the tracer(s) as they will accumulate in active regions of the brain and thus give an indirect measure of changes in neuronal activity.

Postural tremor: tremor that occurs when a part of the body is held voluntarily in a position against gravity. For example, tremor that appears when a patient holds their arms out in front of them.

Postsynaptic: nerve cell that is receiving a signal across a synapse.

Presynaptic: nerve cell that is transmitting the signal across a synapse.

Primidone: barbiturate precursor. GABA agonist used to treat essential tremor.

Propranolol: β-adrenergic blocker—blocks the action of noradrenaline and epinephrine. Used to treat the tremor in essential tremor and, to a lesser degree, Parkinson's disease.

Psychosocial dysfunction: psychological problems in society.

Psychotropic: used to describe drugs that affect (tropic) the mind (psyche). Also called *psychoactive*.

Receptor: part of a protein that binds a specific molecule (ligand). Ligand binding usually activates the receptor protein by changing its shape or function.

Recessive: the inheritance of two copies of a gene defect ($-/-$) is necessary for the manifestation of the phenotype. Heterozygotes ($+/-$) are unaffected.

Rest tremor: tremor that occurs in part of the body that is fully relaxed and completely supported against gravity (e.g. tremor in an arm occurring when the patient is resting on a bed).

Saccadic: small very fast and imperceptible movements of the eyes.

Serotonin: excitatory neurotransmitter.

Single photon emission computerized tomography (SPECT): a scanner that can detect and measure the strength of radioactive emissions (photons) from a radioactively labelled chemical inside the body.

Sociophobia: a fear of society.

Sporadic: occurs infrequently and at irregular intervals, refers here to cases of essential tremor with no family history of essential tremor.

Stem cell: the cell used in high turnover tissues such as bone marrow, skin, gut and the testes to replace more mature differentiated cells that are lost through wear and tear. Capable of self-renewal and differentiation.

Stereotactic: building a three-dimensional image (stereo) by touch (tactic). In brain surgery, the word stereotactic implies using the principle of using an *X, Y* and *Z* co-ordinate system to direct the surgeon rather than by performing surgery under direct vision. A number of different imaging techniques are used to perform stereotactic surgery (see DBS).

Strychnine: highly toxic alkaloid isolated from the seeds of a tree (*Strychnos Nux vomica*). Stimulates the peripheral nervous system to cause muscular spasms and convulsions.

Synapse: contact point between a nerve cell terminal (terminal bouton) and other cells to leave a gap (synaptic cleft).

Teratoma: a very primitive stem cell cancer.

THC [Δ(9)-tetrahydrocannabinol]: a psychoactive drug in *cannabis*.

Thalamotomy: a surgical lesion in the thalamus, usually created by making a small burn or series of small burns with an electric probe.

Topiramate: anti-epeleptic drug, GABA agonist. Used to treat essential tremor.

Transgenic: genetically modified organism. Most commonly used to describe genetically engineered mice.

Tremorogenic: used to describe a chemical agent or drug that causes tremor.

Ventriculography: injection of radio-opaque substance into the two cavities in the middle of the brain—used to image (X-rays) the relative position of other parts of the brain.

9 Resources for patients

Organizations for patients

International Essential Tremor Foundation (IETF) (USA)

PO Box 14005, Lenexa, KS 66285-4005, USA
Freephone: +1-888-387-3667
Telephone: +1-913-341-3880
Fax: +1-913-341-1296
E-mail: staff@essentialtremor.org
Web site: http://www.essentialtremor.org

National Tremor Foundation (NTF) (UK)

Harold Wood Hospital (DSC), Romford, Essex RM3 0BE, UK
Freephone: +44-800-3288046
Telephone: +44-1708-386399
Fax: +44-1708-378032
E-mail: tremorfoundation@aol.com
Web site: http://www.tremor.org.uk

The International Essential Tremor Foundation (IETF, USA) was founded in 1998 and the National Tremor Foundation (NTF, UK) was founded in 1992. Both charities were set up to provide patients and their families with timely, quality information on ET. This is primarily accomplished via the quarterly published newsletters. Each issue contains summaries of ongoing research progress as presented at professional educational meetings, articles about specific aspects of tremor written by ET specialist advisers and their colleagues, and suggestions on coping with the various problems associated with ET, written by specialists in the treatment of ET as well as by patients themselves who have found their own unique solutions. The IETF offers two electronic discussion boards that are readily accessible, one for parents of children with ET and the other aimed at adults.

The IETF also maintains a worldwide referral network of neurological specialists experienced in the clinical care of ET patients. For additional one-to-one support, the IETF assists in the formation of local, independent support groups and has begun a chapter programme.

People seeking additional information about their disorder should contact the IETF office located in Kansas, USA or NTF at Romford, Essex, UK.

The IETF funds scientific research into the nosology, aetiology, pathogenesis, treatment or other topics relevant to ET, but this is largely in order to support existing research funded by other organizations such as the NIH. In general, the IETF funds small research grants up to US$25 000 for a given year.

WE MOVE (Worldwide Education and Awareness for Movement Disorders)

204 W, 84th Street, New York, NY 10024, USA
E-mail: wemove@wemove.org
Web site: http://www.wemove.org

WE MOVE is a not-for-profit organization dedicated to educating and informing patients, professionals and the public about the latest advances, management and treatment options for neurological movement disorders.

poETry
Read some whimsical poems about tremor by Elsie J. Doll (Millwauke, USA). Elsie has set up a free web site for her tongue-in-cheek poems, which were inspired by the experiences told to her by people afflicted with ET. For a light-hearted look at ET, visit: http://www.geocities.com/lc22002/Tremor_Tales.html

Text books

Most of the standard academic and clinical neurology-based textbooks only give a brief mention of ET in spite of the fact that it is the most common movement disorder in humans. To fill this gap in the literature, K. Lyons and R. Pahwa recently (June 2005) published a textbook aimed at specialists working on tremor disorders. The book provides information about the epidemiology, clinical characteristics, and medical and surgical treatment of ET and various tremor disorders. Although this is an invaluable reference book for specialist clinicians, it is probably unsuitable for the average non-medical or scientific lay-person.

Handbook of Essential Tremor and Other Tremor Disorders (Neurological Disease and Therapy) by Kelly E. Lyons and Rajesh Pahwa
Published by Taylor and Francis. Hardcover: US$199.95; GBP 110.00.

Accessing the scientific literature

Because it takes so long to write a book and get it published, textbooks are generally about 12–18 months out of date by the time they appear in the bookshop. For example, more than 80 papers a year are currently being published on ET in the scientific literature, so the inevitable delays in getting a book published represent a serious drawback.

In contrast, papers published in the scientific literature generally take less than 3 months from submission to publication online, and this includes a peer-review process to ensure the scientific quality of each and every publication. Furthermore, once the paper is accepted by a journal, the Abstract, which includes the title, authors and a summary of that paper, appears in electronic database searches. The Abstract offers enough information to get a feel for the 'take home message' of the research presented in the paper and, if needed, the full manuscript can be purchased from the journal that published the manuscript.

A simple method of assessing a considerable amount of the research publications and scientific information about ET is to use the search engine: *Google Scholar* and then perform a search, for example by typing in: *essential tremor*.

A reliable method of accessing the scientific literature about ET is at the National Library of Medicine (NLM) run and maintained by the National Institutes of Health (NIH) on behalf of the US Government. This free electronic database (PubMed; www.ncbi.nlm.nih.gov) covers most if not all research reports in all aspects of the life sciences published in a wide range of reputable specialist scientific journals. This literature gives one a feel for the progress that has and has not been made in understanding and treating ET over the last 45 years.

Devices to help people with essential tremor

Hardware

An assistive mouse adaptor invented by IBM is now available which enables people who have hand tremors to have normal use of a personal computer. IBM has licensed the mouse adaptor to Montrose Secam Limited, a small

British electronics company. The cost of the device is: US$134; GBP 85; Euro
128 and is available from:
Montrose Secam Limited
PO Box 40
Iver, Buckinghamshire SL0 9PZ, UK
Telephone: +44-1753-653125
Fax: +44-1753-670970
E-mail: info@montrosesecam.com
Web site: http://www.montrosesecam.com/index1.html

Software

Computer software (*MouseCage*) is also available, to help facilitate the use of
a computer mouse by people with hand tremors. The software can be
downloaded from: http://www.mousecage.com

The MouseCage software costs: US$29.95; GBP 19.95; Euro 29.95 and is
produced by:
Tunic Software (UK)
Software House
67 Lansbury Avenue
Chadwell Heath RM6 6SD, UK
Telephone: +44-7739-252046
Fax: +44-871-733-5278

10 Selected bibliography

General

Bain, P.G. (2000). Tremor assessment and quality of life measurements. *Neurology* **54**, S26–S29.

Bain, P.G. (2002). The management of tremor. *Journal of Neurology, Neurosurgery and Psychiatry* **72**, Suppl 1, I3–I9.

Bain, P.G., Mally, J., Gresty, M. and Findley, L.J. (1993). Assessing the impact of essential tremor on upper limb function. *Journal of Neurology* **241**, 54–61.

Bain, P.G., Findley, L.J, Atchison, P., Beghari, M., Vidailhet, M., Gresty, M., *et al.* (1993). Assessing tremor severity. *Journal of Neurology, Neurosurgery and Psychiatry* **56**, 868–873.

Critchley, M. (1949). Observations on essential (heredofamilial) tremor. *Brain* **72**, 113–139.

Hardesty, D.E., Maraganore, D.M., Matsumoto, J.Y. and Louis, E.D. (2004). Increased risk of head tremor in women with essential tremor: longitudinal data from the Rochester epidemiology project. *Movement Disorders* **19**, 529–533.

Louis, E.D. (2005). Essential tremor. *Lancet Neurology* **4**, 100–110.

Louis, E.D., Dure, L.S. and Pullman, S. (2001). Essential tremor in childhood: a series of nineteen cases. *Movement Disorders* **16**, 921–923.

Louis, E.D., Applegate, L.M., Borden, S., Moskowitz, C. and Jin, Z. (2005). Feasibility and validity of a modified finger–nose–finger test. *Movement Disorders* **20**, 636–639.

Louis, E.D., Fernadez-Alvarez, E., Dure, L.S., Frucht, S. and Ford, B. (2005). Association between male gender and pediatric essential tremor. *Movement Disorders* **20**, 904–906.

Ondo, W.G., Wang, A., Thomas, M. and Dat Vuong, K. (2005). Evaluating factors that can influence spirography ratings in patients with essential tremor. *Parkinsonism and Related Disorders* **11**, 45–48.

Pahwa, R. and Lyons, K.E. (2003). Essential tremor: differential diagnosis and current therapy. *American Journal of Medicine* **115**, 134–142.

Anxiety

Busenbark, K.L., Nash, J., Nash, S., Hubble, J.P. and Koller, W.C. (1991). Is essential tremor benign? *Neurology* **41**, 1982–1983.

Chatterjee, A., Juewicz, E.C., Applegate, L.M. and Louis E.D. (2004). Personality in essential tremor: further evidence of non-motor manifestations of the disease. *Journal of Neurology, Neurosurgery and Psychiatry* **75**, 958–961.

Gasparini, M., Bonifati, V., Fabrizio, E., Fabbrini, G., Brusa, L., Lenzi, G.L. *et al.* (2001). Frontal lobe dysfunction in essential tremor: a preliminary study. *Journal of Neurology* **248**, 399–402.

Lacritz, L.H., Dewey, R., Giller, C. and Cullum, C.M. (2002). Cognitive functioning in individuals with 'benign' essential tremor. *Journal of the International Neuropsychology Society* **8**, 125–129.

Lombardi, W.J., Woolston, D.J., Roberts, J.W. and Gross, R.E. (2001). Cognitive deficits in patients with essential tremor. *Neurology* **57**, 785–790.

Louis, E.D. (2005). Essential tremor. *Lancet Neurology* **4**, 100–110.

Nemeroff, C.B. (2003). The role of GABA in the pathophysiology and treatment of anxiety disorders. *Psychopharmacology Bulletin* **37**, 133–146.

Roy-Byrne, P.P. (2005). The GABA–benzodiazepine receptor complex: structure, function, and role in anxiety. *Journal of Clinical Psychiatry* **66**, 14–120.

Other symptoms in essential tremor

Dogu, O., Sevim, S., Louis, E.D., Kaleagasi, H. and Aral, M. (2004). Reduced body mass index in patients with essential tremor: a population-based study in the province of Mersin, Turkey. *Archives of Neurology* **61**, 386–389.

Frima, N. and Grunewald, R.A. (2005). Abnormal vibration induced illusion of movement in essential tremor: evidence for abnormal muscle spindle afferent function. *Journal of Neurology, Neurosurgery and Psychiatry* **76**, 55–57.

Gasparini, M., Bonifati, V., Fabrizio, E., Fabbrini, G., Brusa, L., Lenzi, G.L. *et al.* (2001). Frontal lobe dysfunction in essential tremor: a preliminary study. *Journal of Neurology* **248**, 399–402.

Hawkes, C., Shah, M. and Findley, L. (2003). Olfactory function in essential tremor: a deficit unrelated to disease duration or severity. *Neurology* **61**, 871–872.

Helmchen, C., Hagenow, A., Miesner, J., Sprenger, A., Rambold, H., Wenzelburger, R. *et al.* (2003). Eye movement abnormalities in essential tremor may indicate cerebellar dysfunction. *Brain* **126**, 1319–1332.

Ondo, W.G., Sutoon, L., Dat Vuong, K., Lai, D. and Janlovic, J. (2003). Hearing impairment in essential tremor. *Neurology* **61**, 1093–1097.

Stolze, H., Petersen, G., Raethjen, J., Wenzelburger, R. and Deuschl., G. (2001). The gait disorder of advanced essential tremor. *Brain* **124**, 2278–2286.

The brain in essential tremor

Bucher, S.F., Seelos, K.C., Dodel, R.C., Reiser, M. and Oertel, W.H. (1997). Activation mapping in essential tremor with functional magnetic resonance imaging. *Annals of Neurology* **41**, 32–40.

Brodkey, J.A., Tasker, R.R., Hamani, C., McAndrews, M.P., Dostrovsky, J.C. and Lozano, A.M. (2004). Tremor cells in the human thalamus: differences among neurological disorders. *Journal of Neurosurgery* **101**, 43–47.

Ceballos-Baumann, A.O., Boecker, H., Fogel, W., Alesch, F., Bartenstein, P., Conrad, B. *et al.* (2001). Thalamic stimulation for essential tremor activates motor and deactivates vestibular cortex. *Neurology* **56**, 1347–1354.

Hellwig, B., Haussler, S., Lauk, M., Guschlbauer, B., Timmer, J. and Lucking, C.H. (2001). Tremor-correlated cortical activity in essential tremor. *Lancet* **357**, 519–523.

Hellwig, B., Schelter, B., Guschlbauer, B., Timmer, J. and Lucking, C.H. (2003). Dynamic synchronisation of central oscillators in essential tremor. *Clinical Neurophysiology* **114**, 1462–1467.

Hua, S.E. and Lenz, F.A. (2005). Posture-related oscillations in human cerebellar thalamus in essential tremor are enabled by voluntary circuits. *Journal of Neurophysiology* **93**, 117–127.

Hua, S.E., Lenz, F.A., Zirh, T.A., Reich, S.G. and Dougherty, P.M. (1998). Thalamic neuronal activity correlated with essential tremor. *Journal of Neurology, Neurosurgery and Psychiatry* **64**, 273–276.

Jenkins, I.H., Bain, P.G., Colebatch, J.G., Thomson, P.D., Findley, L.J., Frackowiak, R. S., *et al.* (1993). A positron emission tomography study of essential tremor: evidence for overactivity of cerebellar connections. *Annals of Neurology* **34**, 82–90.

Louis, E.D., Shungu, D.C., Chan, S., Mao, X., Jurewicz, E.C. and Watner, D. (2002). Metabolic abnormality in the cerebellum in patients with essential tremor: a proton magnetic resonance spectroscopic imaging study. *Neuroscience Letters.* **333**, 17–20.

Molnar, G.F., Pilliar, A., Lozano, A.M. and Dostrovsky, J.O. (2005). Differences in neuronal firing rate in pallidal and cerebellar receiving areas of the thalamus in patients with Parkinson's disease, essential tremor and pain. *Journal of Neurophysiology* **93**, 3904–4101.

Pinto, A.D., Lang, A.E. and Chen, R. (2003). The cerebellothalamocortical pathway in essential tremor. *Neurology* **60**, 1985–1987.

Wills A.J., Jenkins, I.H., Thompson, P.D., Findley L.J. and Brooks, D.J. (1994). Red nuclear and cerebellar but no olivary activation associated with essential tremor: a positron emission tomographic study. *Annals of Neurology* **36**, 636–642.

Wills A.J., Jenkins, I.H., Thompson, P.D., Findley L.J. and Brooks, D.J. (1995). A positron emission tomography study of cerebral activation associated with essential and writing tremor. *Archives of Neurology* **52**, 299–305.

Genetics

Abbruzzese, G., Pigullo, S., Di Maria, E., Martinelli, P., Barone, P., Marchese, R., *et al.* (2001). Clinical and genetic study of essential tremor in the Italian population. *Neurological Science* **22**, 39–40.

Bain, P.G., Findley, L.J., Thompson, P.D., Gresty, M.A., Rothwell, J.C., Harding, A.E. *et al.* (1994). A study of hereditary essential tremor. *Brain* **117**, 805–824.

Conway, D., Bain, P.G., Warner, T.T., Davis, M.B., Findley, L.J., Thompson, P.D., *et al.* (1993). Linkage analysis with chromosome 9 markers in hereditary essential tremor. *Movement Disorders* **8**, 374–376.

Gulcher, J.R., Jonsson, P., Kong, A., Kristjansson, K., Frigge, M.L., Karason, A., *et al.* (1997). Mapping of a familial essential tremor gene, *FET1* to chromsome 3q13. *Nature Genetics* **17**, 84–87.

Higgins, J.J., Pho, L.T. and Nee, L.E. (1997). A gene (ETM) for essential tremor maps to chromosome 2p22–p25. *Movement Disorders* **12**, 859–864.

Higgins, J.J., Loveless, J.M., Jankovic, J. and Patel, P.I. (1998). Evidence that a gene for essential tremor maps to chromosome 2p in four families. *Movement Disorders* **13**, 972–977.

Higgins, J.J., Jankovic, J., Lombardi, R.Q., Pucilowska, J., Tan, E.K, Ashizawa, T. *et al.* (2003). Haplotype analysis of the ETM2 locus in familial essential tremor. *Neurogenetics* **4**, 185–189.

Higgins, J.J., Lombardi, R.Q., Tan, E.K., Janlovic, J., Pucilowska, J. and Rooney, J.P. (2004). Haplotype analysis of the ETM2 locus in a Singaporean sample with familial essential tremor. *Clinical Genetics* **66**, 353–357.

Higgins, J.J., Lombardi, R.Q., Pucilowska, J. and Ruszczyk, M.U. (2004). Integrated physical map of the human essential tremor gene region (ETM2) on chromosome 2p24.3–p24.2. *American Journal of Medical Genetics* **127B**, 128–130.

Higgins, J.J., Lombardi, R.Q., Pucilowska, J., Jankovic, J., Tan, E.K. and Rooney, J.P. (2005). A variant of the HS1-BP3 gene is associated with familial essential tremor. *Neurology* **64**, 417–421.

Illarioshkin, S.N., Rakhmonov, R.A., Ivanova-Smolenskaia, I.A., Brice, A., Markova, E.D., Miklina, N.I., *et al.* (2002). Molecular genetic analysis of essential tremor. *Genetika* **38**, 1704–1709. (In Russian.)

Kim, J.-H., Cho, Y.-H., Kim, J.-K., Park, Y.-G. and Chang, J.W. (2005). Frequent sequence variation at the ETM2 locus and its association with sporadic essential tremor in Korea. *Movement Disorders* **20**, 1650–1653.

Kovach, M.J., Ruiz, J., Kimonis, K., Mueed, S., Sinha, S., Higgins, C., *et al.* (2001). Genetic heterogeneity in autosomal dominant essential tremor. *Genetics in Medicine* **3**, 197–199.

Lorenz, D., Frederiksen, H., Moises, H., Kopper, F., Deuschl, G. and Christensen, K. (2004). High concordance for essential tremor in monozygotic twins of old age. *Neurology* **62**, 208–211.

Lucotte, G., Lagarde, J.P., Funalot, B. and Sokoloff, P. (2006). Linkage with the Ser9Gly DRD3 polymorphism in essential tremor families. *Clinical Genetics* **69**, 437–440.

Pigullo, S., Di Maria, E., Marcheses, R., Bellone, E., Gulli, R., Scaglione, C., *et al.* (2003). Essential tremor is not associated with a-synuclein gene haplotypes. *Movement Disorders* **18**, 823–826.

Pigullo, S., De Luca, A., Barone, P., Marcheses, R., Bellone, E., Colosimo, A., *et al.* (2004). Mutational analysis of parkin gene by denaturing high-performance liquid chromatography (DHPLC) in essential tremor. *Parkinsonism and Related Disorders* **10**, 357–362.

Tanner, C.M., Goldman, S.M., Lyons, K.E, Aston, D.A., Tetrud, J.W., Welsh, M.D., *et al.* (2001). Essential tremor in twins—an assessment of genetic vs environmental determinants of etiology. *Neurology* **57**, 1389–1391.

Treatment

Bain, P.G. (1997). The effectiveness of treatment for essential tremor. *Neurologist* **3**, 305–321.

Brin, M.F., Lyons, K.E., Doucette, J., Adler, C.H., Caviness, J.N., Comella, C.L., *et al.* (2001). A randomized, double masked, controlled trial of botulinum toxin type A in essential hand tremor. *Neurology* **56**, 1523–1528.

Bushara, K.O., Goldstein, S.R., Grimes, G.J., Burstein, A.H. and Hallett, M. (2004). Pilot trial of 1-octanol in essential tremor. *Neurology* **62**, 122–124.

Calzetti, S., Findley, L.J., Gresty, M.A., Perucca, E. and Richens, A. (1983). Effect of a single dose of propranolol on essential tremor: a double-blind controlled study. *Annals of Neurology* **13**, 165–171.

Carroll, C.B., Bain, P.G., Teare, L., Liu, X., Joint, C., Wroath, C., *et al.* (2004). Cannabis for dyskinesia in Parkinson's disease: a randomized double-blind crossover study. *Neurology* **63**, 1245–1250.

Connor, G.S. (2002). A randomized double-blind placebo controlled trial of topiramate treatment for essential tremor. *Neurology* **59**, 132–134.

Gironell, A., Kulisevsky, J., Barbanoj, M., Lopez-Villegas, D., Hernandez, G. and Pacual-Sedano, B. (1999). A randomized placebo-controlled comparative trial of gabapentin and propranolol in essential tremor. *Archives of Neurology* **56**, 475–480.

Iwat, S., Nomoto, N. and Fukuda, T. (1993). Effects of beta-adrenergic blockers on drug-induced tremors. *Pharmacology, Biochemistry and Behaviour* **44**, 611–613.

Jankovic, J., Schwartz, K., Clemence, W., Aswad, A. and Mordaunt, J. (1996). A randomized, double-blind, placebo-controlled study to evaluate botulinum toxin type A in essential hand tremor. *Movement Disorders* **11**, 250–256.

Larsen, T.A., Teravainen, H. and Calne, D.B. (1982). Atenolol vs propranolol in essential tremor. A controlled quantitative study. *Acta Neurologica Scandinavica* **66**, 547–554.

Ondo, W., Hunter, C., Vuong, K.D., Schwartz, K. and Jankovic, J. (2000). Gabapentin for essential tremor: a multiple-dose, double-blind, placebo-controlled trial. *Movement Disorders* **15**, 678–682.

Ondo, W.G., Jankovic, J., Connor, G.S., Pahwa, R., Elble, R., Stacy, M.A., *et al.* on behalf of the Topiramate Essential Tremor Study Investigators (2006). Topiramate in essential tremor. A double-blind, placebo-controlled trial. *Neurology* **66**, 672–677.

O'Suilleabhain, P. and Dewy, R.B. (2002). Randomized trial comparing primidone initiation schedules for treating essential tremor. *Movement Disorders* **17**, 382–386.

Pahapill, P.A., Levy, R., Dostrvsky, J.O., Davis, K.D., Rezai, A.R., Tasker, R. *et al.* (1999). Tremor arrest with thalamic microinjections of muscimol in patients with essential tremor. *Annals of Neurology* **46**, 249–252.

Pahwa, R., Busenbark, K., Swanson-Hyland, E.F., Dubinsky, R.M., Hubble, J.P., Gray, C. *et al.* (1995). Botulinum toxin treatment of essential head tremor. *Neurology* **45**, 822–824.

Pahwa, R., Lyons, K., Hubble, J.P., Busenbark, K., Rienerth, J.D., Pahwa, A. *et al.* (1998). Double-blind controlled trial of gabapentin in essential tremor. *Movement Disorders* **13**, 465–467.

Serrano-Duenas, M. (2003). Use of primidone in low doses (250 mg/day) versus high doses (750 mg/day) in the management of essential tremor. Double-blind comparative study with one-year follow-up. *Parkinsonism and Related Disorders* **10**, 29–33.

Deep brain stimulation in essential tremor

Benabid, A.L., Benazzous, A. and Pollak, P. (2002). Mechanisms of deep brain stimulation. *Movement Disorders* **17**, S73–S74.

Fields, J.A., Troster, A.I., Woods, S.P., Higginson, C.I., Wilkinson, S.B., Lyons, K.E. *et al.* (2003). Neurophysiological and quality of life outcomes 12 months after unilateral thalamic stimulation for essential tremor. *Journal of Neurology, Neurosurgery and Psychiatry* **74**, 305–311.

Koller, W.C., Lyons, K.E., Wilkinson, S.B. and Pahwa, R. (1999). Efficacy of unilateral deep brain stimulation of the VIM nucleus of the thalamus for essential head tremor. *Movement Disorders* **14**, 847–850.

Krauss, J.K., Simpson, R.K., Ondo, W.G., Pohle, T., Burgunder, J.M. and Jankovic, J. (2001). Concepts and methods in chronic thalamic stimulation for treatment of tremor: technique and application. *Neurosurgery* **48**, 535–541.

Loher, T.J., Gutbrod, K., Fravi, N.L., Pohle, T., Burgunder, J.M. and Krauss, J.K. (2003). Thalamic stimulation for tremor. Subtle changes in episodic memory are related to stimulation *per se* and not to a microthalamotomy effect. *Journal of Neurology* **250**, 707–713.

Lyons, K.E. and Pahwa, R. (2004). Deep brain stimulation and essential tremor. *Journal of Clinical Neurophysiology* **21**, 2–5.

Lyons, K.E., Wilkinson, S.B., Overman, J. and Pahwa, R. (2004). Surgical hardware complications of subthalmic stimulation: a series of 160 procedures. *Neurology* **63**, 612–616.

Obwegeser, A.A., Utti, R.J., Turk, M.F., Strongosky, A.J. and Wharen, R.E. (2000). Thalamic stimulation for the treatment of midline tremors in essential tremor patients. *Neurology* **54**, 2342–2344.

Pahwa, R., Lyons, K.E., Wilkinson, S.B., Troster, A.I., Overman, J., Kieltyka, J. *et al.* (2001). Comparison of thalamotomy to deep brain stimulation of the thalamus in essential tremor. *Movement Disorders* **16**, 140–143.

Papavassiliou, E., Rau, G., Heath, S., Abosch, A., Barbaro, N.M., Larson, P.S., *et al.* (2004). Thalamic deep brain stimulation for essential tremor: relation of lead location to outcome. *Neurosurgery* **54**, 1120–1129.

Plaha, P., Patel, N.K. and Gill, S.S. (2004). Stimulation of the subthalmic region for essential tremor. *Journal of Neurosurgery* **101**, 48–54.

Sydow, O., Thobois, S., Alesch, F., Speelman, J.D. and study collaborators (2003). Multicentre European study of thalamic stimulation in essential tremor: a six year follow up. *Journal of Neurology, Neurosurgery and Psychiatry* **74**, 1387–1391.

Vaillancourt, D.E., Sturman, M.M., Verhagen Metman, L., Bakay, R.A. and Corcos, D.M. (2003). Deep brain stimulation of the VIM thalamic nucleus modifies several features of essential tremor. *Neurology* **61**, 919–925.

Alcohol and essential tremor

Boecker, H., Wills, A.J., Ceballos-Baumann, A., Samuel, M., Thompson, P.D., Findley, L.J. *et al.* (1996). The effect of ethanol on alcohol-responsive essential tremor: a positron emission tomography study. *Annals of Neurology* **39**, 650–658.

Klebe, S., Stolze, H., Grensing, K., Volkmann J., Wenzelburgeer, R. and Deuschl., G. (2005). Influence of alcohol on gait in patients with essential tremor. *Neurology* **12**, 96–101.

Koller, W.C. (1983). Alcoholism in essential tremor. *Neurology* **33**, 1074–1076.

Koob, G.F. (2004). A role for GABA mechanisms in the motivational effects of alcohol. *Biochemical Pharmacology* **68**, 1515–1525.

Nasrallah, H.A., Schroeder, D. and Petty, F. (1982). Alcoholism secondary to essential tremor. *Journal of Clinical Psychiatry* **43**, 163–164.

Rautakorpi, I., Martilla, R.J. and Rinne, U.K. (1983). Alcohol consumption of patients with essential tremor. *Acta Neurologica Scandinavica* **68**, 177–179.

Schroeder, D. and Nasrallah, H.A. (1982). High alcoholism rate in patients with essential tremor. *American Journal of Psychiatry* **139**, 1471–1473.

Zeuner, K.E., Molloy, F.M., Shoge, R.O., Goldstein, S.R., Wesley, R. and Hallett, M. (2003). Effect of ethanol on the central oscillator in essential tremor. *Movement Disorders* **18**, 1280–1285.

Living and coping with essential tremor

Bilodeau, M., Keen, D.A., Sweeney, P.J., Shields, R.W. and Enoka, R.M. (2000). Strength training can improve steadiness in persons with essential tremor. *Muscle and Nerve* **23**, 771–778.

Boulenger, J-P., Uhde, T.W., Wolff, E.A. and Post, R.M. (1984). Increased sensitivity to caffeine in patients with panic disorders. *Archives of General Psychiatry* **41**, 1067–1071.

Hawkes, C., Shah, M. and Findley, L. (2003). Olfactory function in essential tremor: a deficit unrelated to disease duration or severity. *Neurology* **61**, 871–872.

Jacobson, B.H., Winter-Roberts, K. and Gemmell, H.A. (1991). Influence of caffeine on selected manual manipulation skills. *Perceptual and Motor Skills* **72**, 1175–1181.

Watner, D., Jurewicz, E.C. and Louis, E.D. (2002). Survey of essential tremor patients on their knowledge about the genetics of the disease. *Movement Disorders* **17**, 378–381.

The essential tremor mouse

Kralic, J.E., Korpi, E.R., O'Buckley, T.K., Homanics, G.E. and Morrow, A.L. (2002). Molecular and pharmacological characterization of $GABA_A$

receptor α1 subunit knockout mice. *Journal of Pharmacology and Experimental Therapeutics* **302**, 1037–1045.

Kralic, J.E., Wheeler, M., Renzi, K., Ferguson, C., O'Buckley, T.K., Grobin, A.C., *et al.* (2003). Deletion of GABA$_A$ receptor α1 subunit-containing receptors alters responses to ethanol and other anesthetics. *Journal of Pharmacology and Experimental Therapeutics* **305**, 600–607.

Kralic, J.E., Criswell, H.E., Osterman, J.L., O'Buckley, T.K., Wilkie, M.E., Matthews, D.B., *et al.* (2005). Genetic essential tremor in γ-aminobutyric acid$_A$ receptor α1 subunit knockout mice. *Journal of Clinical Investigation* **115**, 774–779.

index